NATIONAL ACADEMIES *Sciences Engineering Medicine*

NATIONAL ACADEMIES PRESS
Washington, DC

Long COVID

Examining Long-Term Health Effects of COVID-19 and Implications for the Social Security Administration

Laura Aiuppa Denning and Erin Hammers Forstag, *Rapporteurs*

Board on Health Care Services

Health and Medicine Division

Proceedings of a Workshop

THE NATIONAL ACADEMIES PRESS 500 Fifth Street, NW
Washington, DC 20001

This activity was supported by contracts between the National Academy of Sciences and the U.S. Social Security Administration. Any opinions, findings, conclusions, or recommendations expressed in this publication do not necessarily reflect the views of any organization or agency that provided support for the project.

International Standard Book Number-13: 978-0-309-69035-5
International Standard Book Number-10: 0-309-69035-8
Digital Object Identifier: https://doi.org/10.17226/26619

This publication is available from the National Academies Press, 500 Fifth Street, NW, Keck 360, Washington, DC 20001; (800) 624-6242 or (202) 334-3313; http://www.nap.edu.

Copyright 2022 by the National Academy of Sciences. National Academies of Sciences, Engineering, and Medicine and National Academies Press and the graphical logos for each are all trademarks of the National Academy of Sciences. All rights reserved.

Printed in the United States of America

Suggested citation: National Academies of Sciences, Engineering, and Medicine. 2022. *Long COVID: Examining long-term health effects of COVID-19 and implications for the Social Security Administration: Proceedings of a workshop*. Washington, DC: The National Academies Press. https://doi.org/10.17226/26619.

The **National Academy of Sciences** was established in 1863 by an Act of Congress, signed by President Lincoln, as a private, nongovernmental institution to advise the nation on issues related to science and technology. Members are elected by their peers for outstanding contributions to research. Dr. Marcia McNutt is president.

The **National Academy of Engineering** was established in 1964 under the charter of the National Academy of Sciences to bring the practices of engineering to advising the nation. Members are elected by their peers for extraordinary contributions to engineering. Dr. John L. Anderson is president.

The **National Academy of Medicine** (formerly the Institute of Medicine) was established in 1970 under the charter of the National Academy of Sciences to advise the nation on medical and health issues. Members are elected by their peers for distinguished contributions to medicine and health. Dr. Victor J. Dzau is president.

The three Academies work together as the **National Academies of Sciences, Engineering, and Medicine** to provide independent, objective analysis and advice to the nation and conduct other activities to solve complex problems and inform public policy decisions. The National Academies also encourage education and research, recognize outstanding contributions to knowledge, and increase public understanding in matters of science, engineering, and medicine.

Learn more about the National Academies of Sciences, Engineering, and Medicine at **www.nationalacademies.org**.

Consensus Study Reports published by the National Academies of Sciences, Engineering, and Medicine document the evidence-based consensus on the study's statement of task by an authoring committee of experts. Reports typically include findings, conclusions, and recommendations based on information gathered by the committee and the committee's deliberations. Each report has been subjected to a rigorous and independent peer-review process and it represents the position of the National Academies on the statement of task.

Proceedings published by the National Academies of Sciences, Engineering, and Medicine chronicle the presentations and discussions at a workshop, symposium, or other event convened by the National Academies. The statements and opinions contained in proceedings are those of the participants and are not endorsed by other participants, the planning committee, or the National Academies.

Rapid Expert Consultations published by the National Academies of Sciences, Engineering, and Medicine are authored by subject-matter experts on narrowly focused topics that can be supported by a body of evidence. The discussions contained in rapid expert consultations are considered those of the authors and do not contain policy recommendations. Rapid expert consultations are reviewed by the institution before release.

For information about other products and activities of the National Academies, please visit www.nationalacademies.org/about/whatwedo.

PLANNING COMMITTEE ON LONG-TERM HEALTH EFFECTS STEMMING FROM COVID-19 AND IMPLICATIONS FOR THE SOCIAL SECURITY ADMINISTRATION

WALTER R. FRONTERA (*Chair*), Professor, Department of Physical Medicine, Rehabilitation and Sports Medicine and Department of Physiology, University of Puerto Rico School of Medicine
ADAORA A. ADIMORA, Sarah Graham Kenan Distinguished Professor of Medicine, Division of Infectious Diseases, University of North Carolina School of Medicine
RANY CONDOS, Clinical Professor, Department of Medicine, New York University Grossman School of Medicine; Director, Post-COVID Program and Adult Cystic Fibrosis Program, NYU Langone Health
STEVEN G. DEEKS, Professor of Medicine in Residence, University of California, San Francisco School of Medicine
ANDREA M. LERNER, Medical Officer, Office of the Director, National Institute of Allergy and Infectious Diseases, National Institutes of Health
MANSOOR A. MALIK, Clinical Professor, Department of Psychiatry and Behavioral Sciences, Johns Hopkins University School of Medicine
LAURA A. MALONE, Physician Scientist, Center for Movement Studies, Kennedy Krieger Institute; Co-director, Pediatric Post–COVID-19 Rehabilitation Clinic, Kennedy Krieger Institute; Assistant Professor, Department of Neurology and Department of Physical Medicine and Rehabilitation, Johns Hopkins University School of Medicine
AVINDRA NATH, Senior Investigator and Clinical Director, Section of Infections of the Nervous System, National Institute of Neurological Disorders and Stroke, National Institutes of Health
MONICA VERDUZCO-GUTIERREZ, Professor and Chair, Department of Rehabilitation Medicine, Joe R. and Teresa Lozano Long School of Medicine, University of Texas Health, San Antonio

Health and Medicine Division Staff

LAURA AIUPPA DENNING, Senior Program Officer
VICTORIA BROWN, Senior Program Assistant
SHARYL NASS, Senior Director, Board on Health Care Services

Consultant

ERIN HAMMERS FORSTAG, Consulting Writer

Reviewers

This Proceedings of a Workshop was reviewed in draft form by individuals chosen for their diverse perspectives and technical expertise. The purpose of this independent review is to provide candid and critical comments that will assist the National Academies of Sciences, Engineering, and Medicine in making each published proceedings as sound as possible and to ensure that it meets the institutional standards for quality, objectivity, evidence, and responsiveness to the charge. The review comments and draft manuscript remain confidential to protect the integrity of the process.

We thank the following individuals for their review of this proceedings:

LIDA BENINSON, National Academies of Sciences, Engineering, and Medicine
SARAH RUIZ, Patient-Centered Outcomes Research Institute
LAURA TABACOF, Icahn School of Medicine at Mount Sinai

Although the reviewers listed above provided many constructive comments and suggestions, they were not asked to endorse the content of the proceedings nor did they see the final draft before its release. The review of this proceedings was overseen by **ALAN M. JETTE,** MGH Institute of Health Professions. He was responsible for making certain that an independent examination of this proceedings was carried out in accordance with standards of the National Academies and that all review comments were carefully considered. Responsibility for the final content rests entirely with the rapporteurs and the National Academies. We also thank staff member Lida Beninson for reading and providing helpful comments on this manuscript.

Acknowledgments

The National Academies of Sciences, Engineering, and Medicine's Board on Health Care Services wishes to express its sincere gratitude to the planning committee chair, Walter Frontera, for his valuable contributions to the development and orchestration of this workshop. The board also wishes to thank all the members of the planning committee, who collaborated to ensure a workshop replete with informative presentations and moderated rich discussions. Finally, the board wants to thank the speakers, who generously shared their expertise and their time with workshop participants. Funding from the Social Security Administration made this workshop possible.

Contents

BOXES, FIGURES, AND TABLES   xiii

ABBREVIATIONS   xv

1   **INTRODUCTION**   1
Structure of the Workshop, 4
Overview of SSA Disability Evaluation, 5

2   **OVERVIEW OF LONG COVID AND DISABILITY**   13
What is Long COVID?, 13
Burden of Disease, 20
Impact of COVID-19 on the Workforce, 25
Discussion, 28

3   **POSTACUTE SEQUELAE OF SARS-COV-2 INFECTION AND IMPLICATIONS FOR RECOVERY**   31
Neurological and Neuromuscular Sequelae, 31
Neuropsychiatric Sequelae, 34
Cardiovascular Sequelae and Autonomic Syndrome, 36
Pulmonary Sequelae, 37
Musculoskeletal, Fatigue, and Pain Sequelae, 39
Discussion, 41

4	**PATIENT AND CAREGIVER PERSPECTIVES ON LIVING WITH LONG COVID**	**45**

Patient Stories, 45
Discussion, 48

5	**LONG-TERM IMPAIRMENTS AND FUNCTIONAL LIMITATIONS RELATED TO LONG COVID**	**53**

Physical Function, Cognitive Function, and Health-Related Quality of Life, 53
Limitations and Impairments after a Stay in the Intensive Care Unit, 57
Mental Health Effects, 62
Child and Adolescent Functioning, 62
ClinFIT COVID-19: A Novel Tool to Assess Functioning, 65
Discussion, 66

6	**CLINICAL PRACTICES AND SYSTEM APPROACHES FOR IMPROVING HEALTH AND RECOVERY FROM LONG COVID**	**73**

Clinical Guidance Statements, 73
Integrated Care Model: Adult Population, 75
Integrated Care Model: Pediatric Population, 77
Overcoming Barriers to Health and Social Inequities, 80
Discussion, 83

7	**EXPLORING FUTURE DIRECTIONS IN THE TREATMENT OF LONG COVID**	**87**

Discussion, 89
Close of Workshop, 92

APPENDIXES
A References 93
B Workshop Agenda 103
C Biographical Sketches of Workshop Planning Committee Members and Speakers 109

Boxes, Figures, and Tables

BOXES

1-1 Statement of Task, 3
1-2 Key Points by Individual Speakers and Participants, 8

FIGURES

2-1 Natural history of SARS-CoV-2 infection, 15
2-2 Body systems affected by SARS-CoV-2 infection, 16
2-3 RECOVER study plan, 19
2-4 Duration of Long COVID among community mild/moderate COVID cases, 22
2-5 Duration of Long COVID among hospitalized COVID cases, 23
2-6 Share of a sector in total loss in employment, 26
2-7 Number of people ages 16 and older with a disability, in thousands, 27
2-8 Percentage of population ages 16 and older that is employed, 28

3-1 Long COVID symptoms, 33

5-1 Full time employment pre- and post-COVID-19, 55
5-2 Neuro QOL Cognitive Function scale scores among patients with postacute COVID-19 infection, 57

xiii

5-3 Health-related quality of life on the EuroQol-5D-5L scale among patients with postacute COVID-19 infection, 58
5-4 Employment status among patients with postacute COVID-19 infection, 59
5-5 COVID-19 pandemic-related factors that could exacerbate physical, cognitive, or mental health impairments, 61
5-6 International Classification of Functioning, Disability, and Health model of functioning and disability, 65

6-1 Specialties available during the initial patient visit in post-COVID clinics, 76
6-2 Algorithm used at Penn Medicine post-COVID clinic for providing care to Long COVID patients, 78
6-3 Characteristics associated with COVID-19 and Long COVID, 82

TABLES

2-1 Probability of Ongoing Symptoms at 3, 6, and 12 Months after Acute COVID-19, 24

5-1 ClinFIT COVID-19 Categories, 67

Abbreviations

AAPM&R	American Academy of Physical Medicine and Rehabilitation
ARDS	acute respiratory distress syndrome
CDC	Centers for Disease Control and Prevention
CDR	continuing disability review
ClinFIT	Clinical Functioning Information Tool
GBD	Global Burden of Disease
ICF	International Classification of Functioning, Disability, and Health
IHME	Institute for Health Metrics and Evaluation
MCAS	mast cell activation syndrome
ME/CFS	myalgic encephalomyelitis/chronic fatigue syndrome
MERS	Middle East respiratory syndrome
MIS-C	multisystem inflammatory syndrome in children
NICE	National Institute for Health and Care Excellence
NIH	National Institutes of Health
PASC	postacute sequelae of COVID-19
PICS	postintensive care syndrome

PM&R	physical medicine and rehabilitation
POTS	postural orthostatic tachycardia syndrome
RECOVER	Researching COVID to Enhance Recovery
SARS	severe acute respiratory syndrome
SSA	Social Security Administration
SSDI	Social Security Disability Insurance Program
SSRI	selective serotonin reuptake inhibitor
WHO	World Health Organization

1

Introduction

On March 21 and 22, 2022, the National Academies of Sciences, Engineering, and Medicine held a virtual workshop titled Long COVID: Examining Long-Term Health Effects of COVID-19 and Implications for the Social Security Administration. The workshop, which was sponsored by the Social Security Administration (SSA), was developed by a planning committee in accordance with the Statement of Task (see Box 1-1).[1] This Proceedings of a Workshop describes the presentations from invited subject matter experts and panel discussions held during the workshop, including responses to questions posed by planning committee members, SSA representatives, and the general public. The speakers, panelists, and workshop participants presented a broad range of information relating to Long COVID and disability; Box 1-2 provides a brief summary of key points made by individual participants. Appendix A contains the reference list, Appendix B contains the workshop agenda, and Appendix C contains short biographical sketches of the workshop planning

---

[1] The planning committee's role was limited to planning the workshop, and the Proceedings of a Workshop was prepared by the workshop rapporteurs as a factual summary of what occurred at the workshop. Statements, recommendations, and opinions expressed are those of individual presenters and participants and are not necessarily endorsed or verified by the National Academies of Sciences, Engineering, and Medicine, and they should not be construed as reflecting any group consensus.

committee members and speakers. The speakers' presentations and the webcast have been archived online.[2]

Research on Long COVID is in the early stages, and the information and guidance stemming from this research is evolving quickly. These proceedings highlight some of the emerging findings from various studies that seek to narrow the knowledge gaps. Workshop speakers provided a snapshot of the science on Long COVID as it relates to functioning and disability. Estimates of the percentage of people who may have Long COVID or who are at risk of developing Long COVID are important to understanding Long COVID's effects on population health, the health system, and the labor force. Much research is focused on defining the prevalence of Long COVID in the U.S. population and on quantifying symptom duration, but the estimates vary widely. One meta-analysis and systematic review (Chen et al., 2022) that included 50 studies reported the prevalence of Long COVID among COVID-19 patients ranged from 9 percent to 81 percent, which the study authors said may be partly attributable to differences in sex, region, study population (e.g., hospitalized versus nonhospitalized patients), and follow-up. Chapter 2 of these proceedings describes one research institute's collaborative efforts to develop prevalence estimates as well as estimates of the burden of disease for Long COVID. However, many questions still remain in this area as well as in other areas of Long COVID research. A consensus definition of Long COVID is needed to overcome barriers to understanding this public health problem.

Walter Frontera, planning committee member and professor of physical medicine and rehabilitation and physiology at the University of Puerto Rico School of Medicine, welcomed participants to the workshop. The purpose of the workshop, he said, was to discuss the most current information available on the long-term effects of COVID-19. The workshop featured subject matter experts and discussions of current and emerging research on the potentially disabling health effects of COVID-19 infection. In particular, presentations explored what is known about the long-term effects of a COVID-19 infection on survivors' function and the possible implications for recovery and disability in the context of SSA's disability programs.

SSA asked the National Academies to host this workshop, said Steve Rollins, acting associate commissioner at the SSA Office of Disability Policy, because it is the SSA's responsibility to provide the most accurate evaluations possible for disability claimants, whether their ability to function is limited by "a well-understood and thoroughly studied impairment or some new condition with unknown mechanisms or uncertain etiologies" such as Long

---

[2] The workshop video can be viewed here: https://www.nationalacademies.org/event/03-21-2022/long-term-health-effects-stemming-from-covid-19-and-implications-for-the-social-security-administration-a-workshop (accessed June 6, 2022).

BOX 1-1
Statement of Task

A planning committee of the National Academies of Sciences, Engineering, and Medicine (the National Academies) will plan and host a 1- to 2-day public workshop that will facilitate a discussion focused on long-term and potentially disabling health effects of COVID-19 infection and survivors' ability to work. The workshop shall include presentations on the functional outcomes for individuals who have contracted and survived COVID-19, as well as medical advances, developments, and research in this area.

The workshop shall feature invited presentations and panel discussions on such topics as:

- An overview of ongoing and upcoming research into the long-term effects of COVID-19;
- How gaps in access to treatment and other racial and ethnic disparities influence health and work outcomes for vulnerable populations;
- The most commonly observed long-term post-COVID impairments, their frequency, and distribution of duration;
- Laboratory or other findings showing patterns of pathology and severity associated with specific symptomology, demographics, physical profiles, or certain comorbidities or genetic markers;
- Patterns of long-term, work-related functional decline observed in adults, their frequency, distribution, and associated signs or laboratory findings;
- Distinct patterns of long-term functional decline observed in children, their frequency, distribution, and associated signs or laboratory findings;
- Effect of vaccine administration on the long-term functional effects of COVID-19 and whether this effect varies between socioeconomic or racial and ethnic groups, in particular vulnerable populations, or based on the specific vaccine used or when in relation to COVID infection it was administered;
- Long-term effects on mental health associated with both the virus itself and the societal impacts of the pandemic response and how those effects vary among adults and children;

continued

> **BOX 1-1 Continued**
>
> - Status of work on describing collections of long-term symptoms as identifiable syndromes (e.g., postacute sequelae of SARS-CoV-2 infection [PASC]);
> - Laboratory or other findings demonstrating variations in functional or long-term effects among different strains of the virus;
> - Recent medical advances, promising research, or new technologies that may alter expected functional outcomes in COVID-19 survivors, and potential advances anticipated in the near future;
> - Potential long-term economic and labor effects of the COVID-19 pandemic and how those effects vary with employment sector or the vocational factors of age, education, and work experience.[a]
>
> The planning committee shall develop the agenda for the workshop sessions, select and invite speakers and discussants, and moderate the discussions. The speakers and discussants shall have the experience and knowledge to discuss the differences experienced by various racial and ethnic populations. A proceeding of the presentations and discussions at the workshop shall be prepared by a designated *rapporteur* in accordance with institutional guidelines.
>
> ---
> [a]42 U.S.C. § 423(d)(2)(A) & 42 U.S.C. § 1382c(a)(3)(B).

COVID. The long-term consequences of COVID-19 infection are being felt by hundreds of thousands of Americans, he said, and people are suffering. For those who are applying for disability benefits, it is the SSA's obligation to "do the best evaluation we can with the knowledge we can gather," said Rollins. To this end, this workshop will inform a better understanding of the symptoms of Long COVID, the populations that it affects, its effect on functioning and quality of life, and the state of current and emerging therapies and treatments.

STRUCTURE OF THE WORKSHOP

Frontera gave participants an overview of the structure of the workshop. In the first session, the expert panel set the foundation of the workshop by providing an overview of Long COVID, including how it is diagnosed, the population affected, major research initiatives, and how the pandemic has affected the labor force. The second session delved more deeply into the disabling late effects of Long COVID in adults and children. Session three featured firsthand accounts of Long COVID from five individuals who shared their stories of illness, recovery, and the effect of Long COVID on their lives. The fourth session featured presentations on how function can be assessed in Long COVID survivors and what is known about the effect of COVID-19 on functioning and quality of life in adults and children. In the fifth session, speakers discussed clinical practices and system approaches for improving treatment for Long COVID, as well as approaches for overcoming barriers to inequities in Long COVID care. Finally, said Frontera, the sixth session explored the state of the science on treatment interventions and therapies for Long COVID. In this final session, workshop speakers offered their key insights and messages. This Proceedings of a Workshop follows the structure of the workshop.

OVERVIEW OF SSA DISABILITY EVALUATION

As background for workshop participants who were not familiar with SSA's disability programs, Vincent Nibali, policy analyst at the SSA Office of Disability Policy, provided an overview. SSA administers two programs that provide benefits on the basis of disability, he said: the Social Security Disability Insurance Program (SSDI), and the Supplemental Security Income Program (SSI). Although these two programs have different nonmedical requirements for eligibility, said Nibali, both programs share the same medical criteria and go through the same sequential evaluation processes to determine initial eligibility.

For adults, said Nibali, disability is defined by statute as "inability to do any substantial gainful activity by reason of any medically determinable physical or mental impairment," which can be expected to result in death or last for a continuous period of not less than 12 months (C.F.R. § 404.1505).[3]

---

[3] The definition of disability is described in Section 223(d)(1) of the Social Security Act as an "inability to engage in any substantial gainful activity by reason of any medically determinable physical or mental impairment which can be expected to result in death or which has lasted or can be expected to last for a continuous period of not less than 12 months, or in the case of an individual who has attained the age of 55 and is blind (within the meaning of blindness as defined in section 216(i)(1)), inability by reason of such blindness to engage in substantial gainful activity requiring skills or abilities comparable to those of any gainful activity in which the individual has previously engaged with some regularity and over a substantial period of time" (Social Security Act, 42 U.S.C. § 423(d)).

Nibali noted that the "continuous period of not less than 12 months," is called the "duration requirement," and it has likely implications for the discussions at this workshop. While there are many people who report symptoms at 3 or 6 months following an acute COVID-19 illness, SSA is most interested in information about symptoms that persist for at least 12 months, and whether there is any correlation between markers of acute COVID-19 illness and the persistence of certain symptoms over time.

For children, a finding of disability is based upon having "marked and severe functional limitations" attributable to physical or mental impairments that are expected to cause death or last for a continuous period of at least 12 months (C.F.R. § 416.906). For both children and adults, said Nibali, the outcome of a disability evaluation depends upon the severity of functional limitations arising from the person's impairment or combination of impairments, either because those functional limitations preclude work, or because they are marked and severe. SSA's sequential evaluation processes use a series of specific questions to determine eligibility; these questions are designed to allow adjudicators to decide the clearest cases quickly. For example, Nibali said, the process starts by asking whether the person is engaged in substantial gainful activity; if the answer is yes, the person is not eligible. If the answer is no, the process continues in order to determine if the person has a medically determinable impairment that is severe and meets the duration requirement—that is, if the evidence shows an impairment that has more than a minimal effect on functioning. The third step, said Nibali, captures the most severe and obvious cases of disability by comparing a claimant's impairments against the criteria in the SSA listing of impairments. If the individual meets these requirements, he or she is immediately considered disabled and eligible. If not, the adjudicator continues with the sequential evaluation process to a more in-depth functional analysis to determine the capacity of the individual to perform work, called "residual functional capacity." This capacity is compared against the demands of past work of the individual, and against the work that exists in substantial numbers in the national economy.

Nibali emphasized the absence of Long COVID in the SSA listing of impairments does not mean that individuals will not be eligible for disability benefits, it simply means that the process moves forward to the functional analysis. Nibali said that SSA is interested in hearing about the potential for identifying Long COVID-related criteria that preclude work in all cases; including these in the listings would enable SSA's rapid adjudication of some claims related to COVID-19.

In addition to evaluating initial eligibility, SSA is also tasked with identifying individuals who are no longer eligible for disability benefits, said Nibali. To capture this group, SSA regularly conducts continuing disability reviews (CDRs). The frequency of CDRs is based in part on how likely it is that an individual's underlying impairments will improve over time. This is another area, said Nibali, in which the workshop presentations may be of critical assistance, because the existing information on recovery from Long COVID is minimal. Nibali closed by stating, "A greater understanding of the long-term effects of COVID-19 can contribute to our agency's mission to provide the most accurate disability decisions as efficiently as possible."

BOX 1-2
Key Points by Individual Speakers and Participants[a]

Definition of Long COVID

- Terms used to describe long-lasting symptoms after an acute COVID-19 infection include Long COVID, postacute sequelae of COVID-19 (PASC), and post-COVID condition. (Katz)
- There is no universal clinical case definition for long COVID. Symptoms that are present more than 4 weeks postinfection is the cutoff CDC uses to define Long COVID; the WHO defines it using a period of 3 months from the onset of COVID-19 with symptoms. Currently no strong data support the use of one definition versus another. (Katz, Vos)

Symptoms

- The risk of ongoing symptoms after an acute COVID-19 infection is considerable, especially in young adults and females. Long COVID occurs even in patients with mild infections. Recovery for the vast majority of long COVID cases occurs within a year. (Vos)
- Long COVID is associated with multisystem dysfunction affecting the cerebrovascular, autonomic, peripheral, respiratory, and inflammatory systems, which may be caused by low-grade inflammation that is either systemic or targets the vascular system. (Novak)
- Common post-COVID symptoms are fatigue, headache, brain fog, shortness of breath, hair loss, pain, insomnia, dizziness, memory loss, and palpitations. (Katz, Tabacof, Vos)
- The severity of the symptoms experienced by some patients with Long COVID is similar to the severity of symptoms experienced by patients with other disabling conditions, including postural orthostatic tachycardia syndrome (POTS), myalgic encephalomyelitis/chronic fatigue syndrome, and small fiber neuropathy. (Novak, Komaroff)
- Musculoskeletal disease and symptoms, fatigue, postexertional malaise, and pain often persist for at least 6 months following acute COVID-19. (Komaroff)
- COVID-19 infection is associated with the exacerbation of and new-onset psychiatric disorders, including mood, anxiety, and trauma-related disorders, as well as sleep disturbances. (Kurylo, Troyer)

- In children, the prevalence of Long COVID seems to be lower than in adults, but the sequelae in children following COVID-19 infection is less well understood compared to adults. Children can experience significant long-term physical, cognitive, social, and emotional limitations because of Long COVID. (Johnston, Troyer)

Diagnosis, Assessment, and Treatment

- Guidance for health care professionals will evolve as the evidence about the etiology, assessment, and risks for Long COVID emerges. (Flanagan, Katz, Tabacof, Vázquez, Vos)
- Many clinicians lack an understanding of Long COVID. Variety and variability of symptoms make it challenging to recognize and diagnose Long COVID. Education and training are needed to help clinicians diagnose Long COVID and deliver appropriate patient care. (Katz, Lewis, Tabacof, Vázquez)
- Patient health and well-being can be compromised when their symptoms are not taken seriously, or are misdiagnosed, by medical professionals. (Berger, Denaults, Katz, Lewis, Vázquez, Vos)
- COVID-19 infection is a necessary precursor to Long COVID; however, many patients have not received a confirmatory positive COVID test because of the lack of available tests, particularly early in the pandemic. (Katz, Tabacof, Vázquez)
- Currently, no laboratory or imaging findings provide a definitive diagnosis of Long COVID. Diagnosis requires patient-reported symptoms and outcomes, and clinical evaluation and selective testing based on symptoms. (Deeks, Katz, Novak, Tabacof)
- Evaluation of patients with respiratory complications from COVID-19 can include chest imaging, pulmonary function tests, CT scans, walk tests, and echocardiogram. (Parker)
- Clinical measures to assess functioning in Long COVID patients, such as physical and cognitive stamina on repetitive challenges, are important and available. (Deeks, Komaroff, Stucki)
- There are studies indicating that symptoms such as shortness of breath and fatigue in Long COVID patients may respond well to exercise interventions; however, more research is needed on optimal physical activity and exercise regimens. (Frontera)

continued

BOX 1-2 Continued

- Few COVID-19-specific therapeutic options exist, so treatments for Long COVID symptoms are based on what is known about related conditions, for example, asthma (Parker) or POTS (Novak).

Functional Outcomes

- Functional impairment attributed to Long COVID symptoms is common. Long COVID affects a broad spectrum of functioning domains, ranging from body functions to activities and participation. (Komaroff, Novak, Stucki)
- Long COVID can reduce patient functioning and participation for longer than 12 months, regardless of the severity of acute COVID-19 illness. (Tabacof, Vos)
- Impairments are comparable or more severe than what is seen in other work-debilitating conditions. (Tabacof)
- Debilitating symptoms, which can wax and wane, create uncertainty and unpredictability in all aspects of a patient's life, making it difficult to care for oneself and family, work, go to school, and maintain social connections. Many people face financial challenges as result of loss of income and the cost of care. (Denaults, Lewis, Taylor, Vázquez)
- Pandemic-related factors can place COVID-19 patients who were in the ICU at greater risk for physical, cognitive, or mental health impairments; limitations on activity; or restrictions on social participation, and thus be at higher risk of long-term disability. (Azola)
- In children, early recognition and treatment of symptoms and support of return to school and other activities with appropriate accommodations is essential to the overall recovery. (Johnston, Morrow)
- Identification of family stressors (e.g., financial, housing, employment, safety, social isolation) and availability of support systems may provide emotional and logistical support and guide medical therapies. (Johnston)

Employment and Workforce

- The majority of Long COVID cases are in people of working age. (Vos)
- In the population of people without disabilities, the share employed is still several percentage points lower than in

2019, while in the population of people with disabilities, the share employed has nearly returned to prepandemic levels. (Kochhar)
- Cognitive, mood, and trauma-related symptoms were common among survivors of past coronavirus outbreaks, and nearly a quarter of survivors had not returned to work 3 years postillness. (Troyer)

Societal and Health System Factors

- Social determinants such as poverty, and structural inequalities such as racism and discrimination, increase the risk of acquiring COVID-19 and strongly influence long-term sequelae of COVID-19 and access to care. (Berger, Nath, Troyer)
- Considerable patient support (e.g., rehabilitation, income) and investment in the care delivery infrastructure (e.g., workforce) may help individuals with Long COVID transition back into the workforce. (Tabacof, Vos)
- Integrated, multidisciplinary, team-based approaches have potential to improve the care of children and adults with Long COVID. Numerous integrated care models have been implemented, but work is needed to determine optimal models of clinical care for these patients. (Abramoff, Deeks, Morrow)
- In the field of rehabilitation, making specialized clinics available to smaller hospitals via telehealth may help improve access and reduce disparities in care. (Frontera)
- Important policy priorities include strengthening primary care, optimizing data quality, and address domains of inequity. (Berger)
- The scale of the pandemic will require that brain and mental health be integral components of research and clinical and social service planning in the coming years. (Troyer)

Research

- NIH's RECOVER initiative is designed to increase understanding of Long COVID and provide information to develop new diagnostic tests and treatment approaches for Long COVID. (Katz)
- Longer-term outcomes, pathogenic mechanisms, biomarkers, and effective treatments for post-COVID-19 psychiatric disorders remain to be elucidated. (Troyer)

continued

BOX 1-2 Continued

- There is a need to understand the effects of specific variants of COVID-19 on the development of Long COVID. (Deeks)
- Interventional studies on drugs, biologics, rehabilitation interventions, medical devices, and complementary and alternative therapies are underway. (Deeks)
- Further research aimed at understanding the long-term effect of Long COVID on children as they transition into adulthood is greatly needed. (Johnston)

---

[a] This list is the rapporteurs' summary of points made by the individual speakers identified, and the statements have not been endorsed or verified by the National Academies of Sciences, Engineering, and Medicine. They are not intended to reflect a consensus among workshop participants.

2

Overview of Long COVID and Disability

Frontera introduced the first panel of the workshop, in which speakers gave an overview of Long COVID and disability. These presentations, he said, were designed to explain the symptoms and mechanisms of Long COVID, to describe the burden of disease associated with Long COVID, and to explore the labor market trends during the COVID-19 pandemic. Following the presentations, Frontera moderated a panel discussion to further explore these topics.

WHAT IS LONG COVID?

Stuart Katz, professor of medicine and principal investigator for the RECOVER Clinical Science Core at New York University Langone Health, began the session by giving an overview of what is known about Long COVID, including the variety of symptoms, how it is recognized in clinical practice, and the risk factors for developing Long COVID. There are several terms used to refer to Long COVID, said Katz. The term *Long COVID* was initially coined and popularized by patient advocacy groups to describe long-lasting symptoms after an acute COVID-19 infection. The National Institutes of Health (NIH) introduced the term *postacute sequelae of COVID-19* (PASC) to encompass the total health impact of COVID-19 over time, while the World Health Organization (WHO) and the Centers for Disease Control and Prevention (CDC) use the phrase *post-COVID condition* as an alternative to PASC. In addition, said Katz, a specific and rare type of Long COVID in children is multisystem inflammatory syndrome in children (MIS-C).

Long COVID Symptoms

Katz shared a figure that describes the natural history of SARS-CoV-2 infection (Figure 2-1).[1] The acute phase lasts around 2 weeks for most people; during this time, fever and upper respiratory symptoms are common. A subgroup of people continue to experience symptoms after this initial phase; Katz said symptoms more than 4 weeks postinfection is the cutoff that is generally used to define Long COVID. At that point, these symptoms may be subacute, ongoing symptoms of the infection, or may become chronic, postinfection symptoms that can persist for months or years. The symptoms can affect a number of body systems and organs, from lungs and heart to joints and muscles.

Katz explained that SARS-CoV-2 has a unique mechanism of action; it enters the body through a receptor called angiotensin-converting enzyme 2, or ACE2, that is present in nearly all systems in the body, including the heart, brain, spleen, liver, blood vessels, gastrointestinal tract, kidneys, pancreas, and lungs (Figure 2-2). SARS-CoV-2 enters the body and begins to replicate in multiple systems, causing diverse symptoms and organ dysfunction. In acute COVID-19, said Katz, the lungs are the organs that are most prominently affected, but there are reports of dysfunction across organ systems in both acute and chronic phases.

In 2021, a systematic review of studies assessing long-term effects of COVID-19 (Lopez-Leon et al., 2021) identified more than 50 symptoms that can be present following an acute COVID-19 infection, including:

- Fatigue (58 percent)
- Headache (44 percent)
- Attention disorder (27 percent)
- Hair loss (25 percent)
- Dyspnea[2] (24 percent)
- Ageusia[3] (23 percent)
- Anosmia[4] (21 percent)
- Postactivity polypnea[5] (21 percent)
- Joint pain (19 percent)
- Cough (19 percent)
- Sweat (17 percent)

---

[1] The novel coronavirus, or SARS-CoV-2, is the virus that causes COVID-19 disease.
[2] Shortness of breath.
[3] Loss of sense of taste.
[4] Loss of sense of smell.
[5] Rapid breathing.

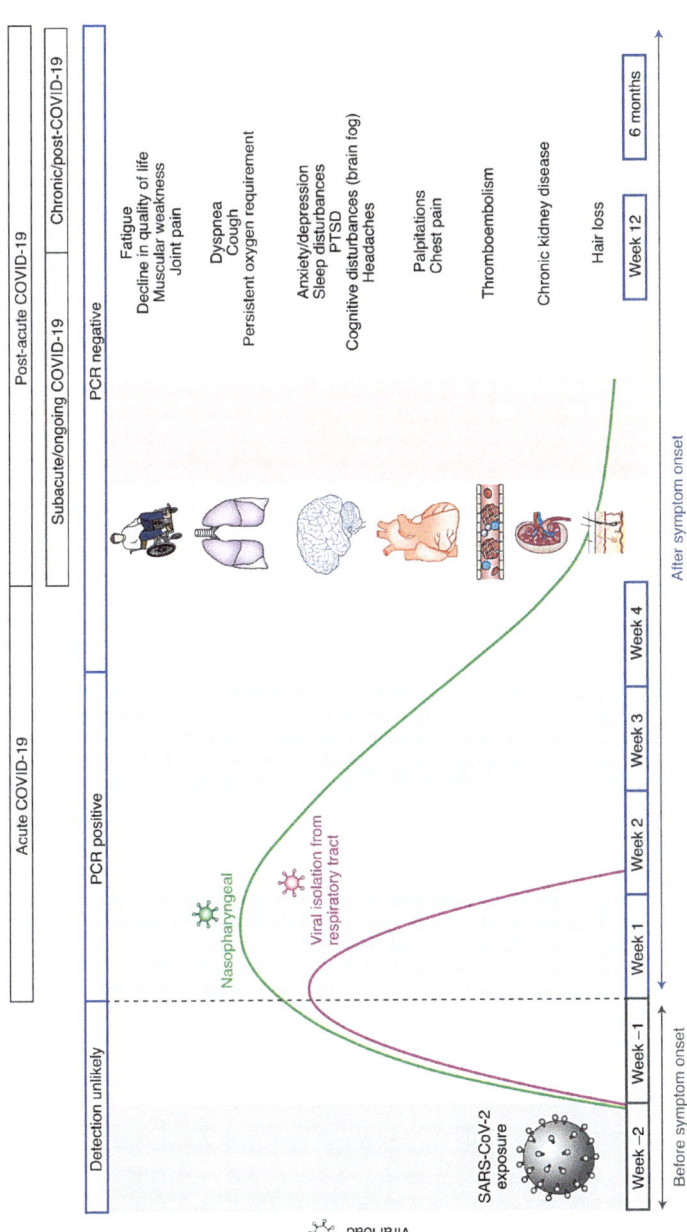

FIGURE 2-1 Natural history of SARS-CoV-2 infection.
SOURCE: Reprinted by permission from Springer Nature, Nature Medicine 27(4), Nalbanian et al., 2021, p. 602, in Stuart Katz presentation, March 21, 2022.

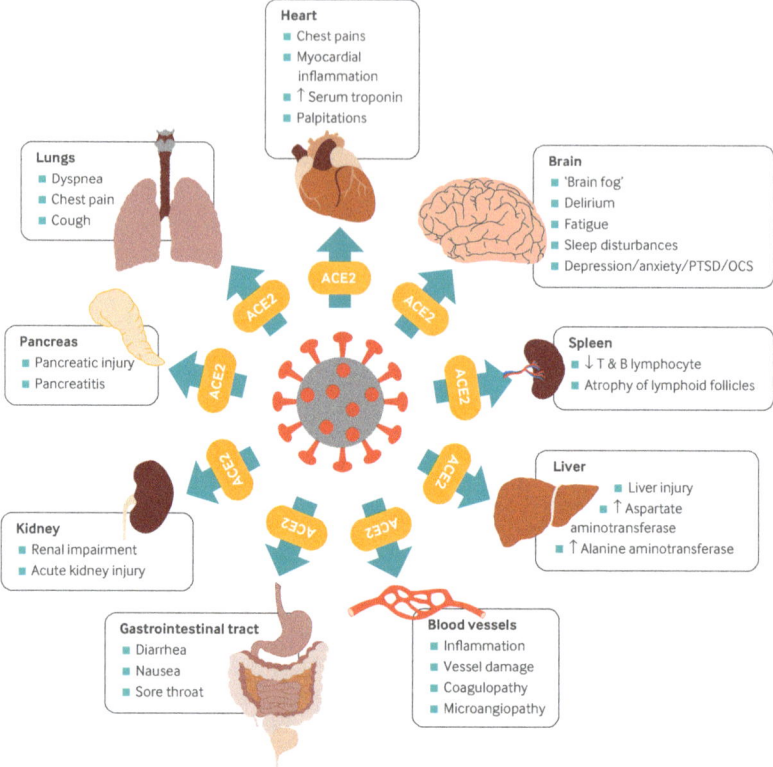

FIGURE 2-2 Body systems affected by SARS-CoV-2 infection.
NOTE: ACE2 = angiotensin-converting enzyme 2; PTSD = posttraumatic stress disorder; OCS = obsessive compulsive spectrum disorders.
SOURCE: Reproduced from Crook et al., 2021, p. 2, with permission from BMJ Publishing Group Ltd., in Stuart Katz presentation, March 21, 2022.

- Memory loss (16 percent)
- Nausea or vomit (16 percent)
- Chest pain or discomfort (16 percent)
- Hearing loss or tinnitus (15 percent)

Katz noted that while many people may occasionally experience some of these symptoms in everyday life, particularly fatigue, Long COVID patients report that it is an "unnatural type of fatigue" that prevents them from performing normal activities and does not improve with increased rest. The review study (Lopez-Leon et al., 2021) found that 80 percent of people report at least one symptom after the acute phase of COVID-19 and that the range of symptoms involved virtually every organ system. Data on how long post-COVID symptoms last are limited, said Katz. One study used a smartphone app to collect survey data and compare persons who tested positive with those who tested negative; those persons who tested positive were more likely to have symptoms persisting at 28 and 56 days following the onset of infection (Sudre et al., 2021). Katz noted that survey participants were young and ambulatory, so their experience may not be representative of the general population. Evidence on post-COVID symptoms, said Katz, demonstrates that symptoms can wax and wane over time. For some patients, symptoms may start during the acute phase and continue into the chronic phase; other patients may feel fully recovered after acute COVID-19 and begin to experience symptoms weeks or months after the infection. The mix of symptoms may vary over time as well, for example, a patient's breathing may improve at the same time that their brain fog (difficulty concentrating) is increasing.

The variety and variability of symptoms make it challenging to recognize and diagnose Long COVID. There is no established diagnostic test for the transition from acute COVID-19 to Long COVID; some markers of inflammation from acute infection have been found to persist at least 28 days, said Katz. While COVID-19 infection is a necessary precursor to Long COVID, some patients lacked access to definitive testing, particularly in the early days of the pandemic.

Definitions of Long COVID

Because the science is incomplete at this time, Katz noted that the definition of Long COVID is variable and "arbitrary." For example, some sources use a 3-month threshold from the date of acute COVID-19 onset (WHO, 2021), others use a 4-week threshold (CDC, 2021b), and still others define it differently (Haute Autorité de Santé, France, 2021; Nalbandian et al., 2021; NICE, 2020; Royal Society, 2020).

The WHO conducted a consensus-building exercise to develop a definition of Long COVID, said Katz; it reads:

> Post COVID-19 condition occurs in individuals with a history of probable or confirmed SARS-CoV-2 infection, usually 3 months from the onset of COVID-19 with symptoms and that last for at least 2 months and cannot be explained by an alternative diagnosis. Common symptoms include fatigue, shortness of breath, cognitive dysfunction, but also others and generally have an impact on everyday functioning. Symptoms may be new onset following initial recovery from an acute COVID-19 episode or persist from the initial illness. Symptoms may also fluctuate or relapse over time. (WHO, 2021, p. 1)

In the United States, the CDC uses the umbrella term *post-COVID conditions* to encompass the "wide range of physical and mental health consequences experienced by some patients that are present 4 or more weeks after SARS-CoV-2 infection, including by patients who had initial mild or asymptomatic acute infection" (CDC, 2021b). Katz quoted the CDC guidance concerning the diagnosis of post-COVID conditions, which states:

> Objective laboratory or imaging findings should not be used as the only measure or assessment of a patient's well-being; lack of laboratory or imaging abnormalities does not invalidate the existence, severity, or importance of a patient's symptoms or conditions. (CDC, 2021b)

Further, the CDC guidance states: "Understanding of post-COVID conditions remains incomplete, and guidance for health care professionals will likely change over time as the evidence evolves."

Long COVID Research

While evidence is still evolving, a number of risk factors can make it more likely that an individual will develop Long COVID, said Katz. These include a greater number of symptoms during the acute phase of COVID-19 infection, severe acute symptoms, hospitalization owing to COVID-19, and preexisting comorbidities. The effects of race, ethnicity, vaccination status, and different variants of SARS-CoV-2 on developing Long COVID are still uncertain.

Katz told workshop participants about a National Institutes of Health (NIH) research initiative to learn more about Long COVID. RECOVER (Researching COVID to Enhance Recovery) is a multisite observational study designed to increase understanding of the epidemiology and mechanisms of Long COVID,[6] said Katz. The study aims to answer a number of questions:

- How many people are getting Long COVID?
- Why do some people get Long COVID and others do not?
- What symptoms do people feel when they get Long COVID?
- How long do people feel sick when they get Long COVID?
- What causes Long COVID to occur?

The RECOVER study includes people with and without a history of COVID-19, and uses cohorts that include pregnant women and their infants, children, and adults. Participants may be enrolled at the time of acute COVID-

---

[6] More information about RECOVER can be found at https://www.recovercovid.org (accessed May 7, 2022).

19 infection or at any time after an infection. This design, said Katz, allows the study to collect information across the different variants and from different times of the pandemic. Participant recruitment is planned in all 50 states, and the study aims to enroll a diverse population that matches the impact of COVID-19 in the United States. Katz noted that NIH awarded RECOVER grants to sites that demonstrate strong connections to local communities and the ability to enroll diverse populations. In addition, RECOVER has both a national community engagement group and a community engagement toolbox to facilitate interaction with the sites.

RECOVER uses a tiered approach (Figure 2-3) that begins with screening tests of 40,000 participants; the screening examines symptoms, risk of PASC after COVID-19, and how pandemic-related stress may affect PASC. The second tier includes participants with symptoms (and appropriate healthy controls for comparison); this group of 10,000 will undergo additional testing. Finally, a smaller subgroup of 4,500 will undergo additional, more in-depth testing to gain insight into the mechanisms of PASC. In addition, the study integrates electronic health record data; Katz said that using these "real-world" data can help us understand the ways PASC affects people's lives and support the development of new diagnostic tests and therapeutic targets.

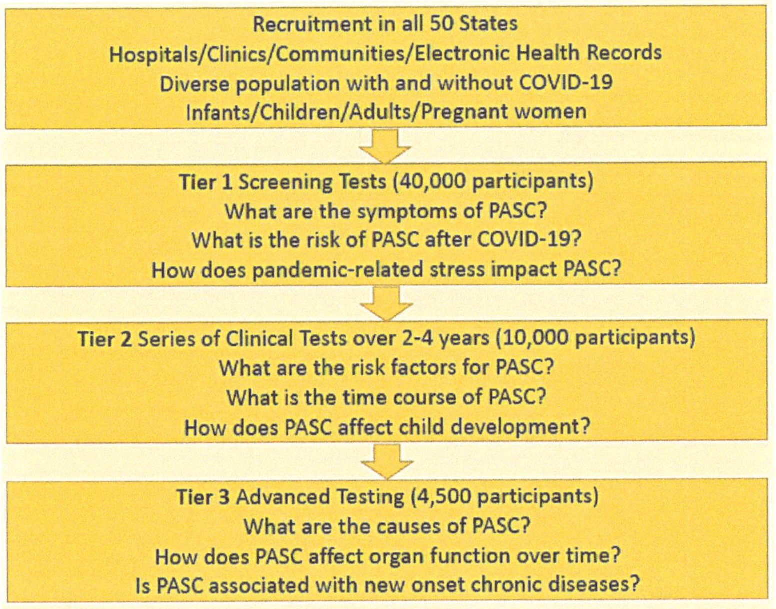

Recruitment in all 50 States
Hospitals/Clinics/Communities/Electronic Health Records
Diverse population with and without COVID-19
Infants/Children/Adults/Pregnant women

⬇

Tier 1 Screening Tests (40,000 participants)
What are the symptoms of PASC?
What is the risk of PASC after COVID-19?
How does pandemic-related stress impact PASC?

⬇

Tier 2 Series of Clinical Tests over 2-4 years (10,000 participants)
What are the risk factors for PASC?
What is the time course of PASC?
How does PASC affect child development?

⬇

Tier 3 Advanced Testing (4,500 participants)
What are the causes of PASC?
How does PASC affect organ function over time?
Is PASC associated with new onset chronic diseases?

FIGURE 2-3 RECOVER study plan.
NOTE: PASC = postacute sequelae of COVID-19.
SOURCE: Stuart Katz presentation, March 21, 2022.

In closing, Katz summarized the main points of his presentation:

- Long COVID is an umbrella term for the wide range of physical and mental health consequences experienced by some patients that are present 4 or more weeks after SARS-CoV-2 infection.
- The most common post-COVID symptoms are fatigue, headache, brain fog, shortness of breath, hair loss, and pain.
- Understanding of post-COVID conditions remains incomplete, and guidance for health care professionals will likely change as the evidence evolves.
- NIH's RECOVER initiative is designed to increase understanding of Long COVID and provide information to develop new diagnostic tests and treatment approaches for Long COVID.

BURDEN OF DISEASE

Early in the COVID-19 pandemic, the focus was on managing acute infections, preventing spread, and tracking case rates and deaths, said Theo Vos, professor of health metrics sciences at the Institute for Health Metrics and Evaluation (IHME) at the University of Washington. As the pandemic continued, reports of long-term symptoms began to surface. Many studies concentrated simply on identifying and listing symptoms, and there was no systematic approach to measuring symptom severity. Vos and his colleague, Sarah Wulf Hanson, research scientist at IHME at the University of Washington, set out to create a systematic approach for making epidemiologic estimates for Long COVID, with the aim of adding Long COVID to the Global Burden of Disease (GBD) estimates, which quantify health loss from diseases, injuries, and risk factors.[7] Vos shared their preliminary estimates of Long COVID with workshop participants, noting that the estimates would soon be finalized and available following the workshop (see Hanson et al., 2022, for the final results).

Limitations of what could be derived from existing publications led him and Hanson to seek opportunities to collaborate with ongoing cohort studies in order to draw a more comprehensive picture of Long COVID. Vos and Hanson gained access to the individual records from 10 cohort studies from around the world, medical claims data in the United States, and data from 40 published sources. Vos said the focus is on three symptom clusters that affect a large proportion of patients: (1) fatigue, body pain, and depression/anxiety; (2) cognitive problems such as inability to concentrate or remember; and (3) ongoing respiratory problems. In each of these categories, the researchers

---

[7] More information about GBD can be found at https://www.healthdata.org/gbd/2019 (accessed June 10, 2022).

assigned different GBD disability weights depending on symptom severity. Vos noted that the estimates did not include the added risk of diseases already measured separately in GBD estimates (e.g., cardiovascular disease, kidney disease), and that the researchers made the assumption that asymptomatic infection does not lead to Long COVID. Vos discussed the rationale for this assumption later during the discussion.

Vos presented a selection of their preliminary findings. The first was an estimate of the duration of Long COVID, estimated separately for community cases and hospitalized cases. The median duration for those with mild/moderate infections was 121.5 days from 3 months after symptom onset (Figure 2-4), and the median duration for those who were hospitalized was 268.9 days from 3 months after symptom onset (Figure 2-5).

For people with symptoms that persisted beyond 3 months, Long COVID is more common in adults than children, more common in adult females than adult males, and more common in those who were hospitalized than those who were not. However, a great deal of heterogeneity exists in the studies, so these data have a large uncertainty interval. Using these data on recovery from COVID-19, Vos and Hanson ran models to develop estimates of the likelihood of experiencing Long COVID, based on a variety of factors. The probability of continuing to experience symptoms is greatest at 3 months, decreases over time, and varies by community, hospital, or intensive care unit COVID cases (Table 2-1). Vos noted there are considerable differences in risk between females and males, and while children have a lower probability of Long COVID, it is "far from trivial."

Given these probabilities for ongoing symptoms, and the number of people infected with COVID-19 in the United States in 2020 and 2021, Vos and Hanson estimated the number of new cases of Long COVID in the United States. They estimated about 4.6 million[8] new cases of Long COVID in the United States in 2020 and 2021, he said, using a minimum duration threshold of 3 months after an acute COVID-19 infection. One lesson from these estimates, said Vos, is that the vast majority of people who develop Long COVID had mild infections (86 percent). While the risk of developing Long COVID is lower for those with mild infections, the sheer number of mild infections makes this number quite high overall. Using disability weights, Vos and his colleagues estimate that on average, people lost 21 percent of their health while living in a state of Long COVID. This is equivalent, he said, to the disability weight of people with complete hearing loss or severe traumatic brain injury. For symptoms that persist beyond a year, Vos said the estimate is about 1.4 million[9] cases of Long COVID. This distribution tilts slightly more

---

[8] The speaker updated this number after the presentation.
[9] The speaker updated this number after the presentation.

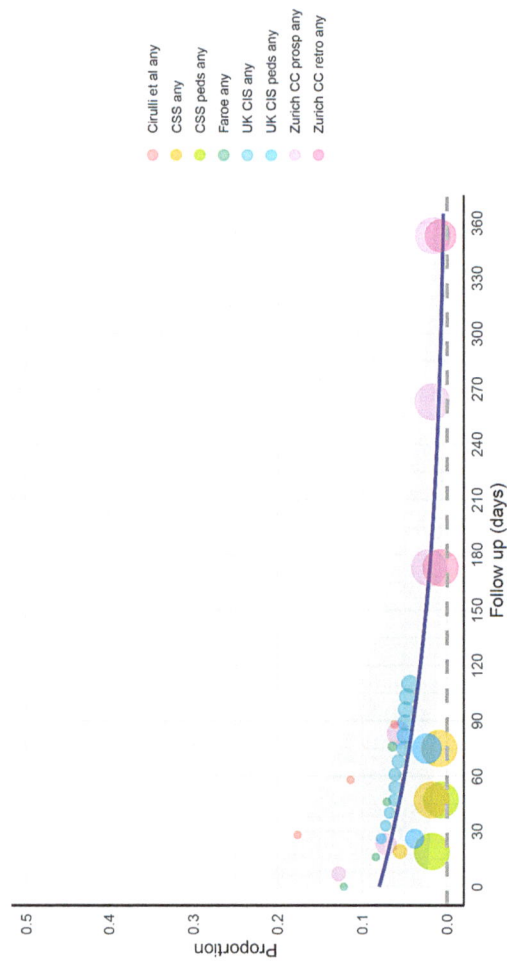

FIGURE 2-4 Duration of Long COVID among community mild/moderate COVID cases.[1]

[1] The speaker updated this figure after the presentation.

NOTE: Cirulli et al any = Cirulli et al., 2020; CSS any = Sudre et al., 2021; CSS peds any = Molteni et al., 2021; Faroe any = Petersen et al., 2021; UK CIS any = UK CIS, 2021, and Ayoubkhani et al., 2021; UK CIS peds = Pediatric population in UK CIS, 2021, and Ayoubkhani et al., 2021; Zurich CC prosp any = Prospective population in Puhan et al., 2021; Zurich CC retro any = Retrospective population in Puhan et al., 2021.
SOURCE: Hanson et al., 2022, Appendix 1, p. 42, in Theo Vos presentation, March 21, 2022.

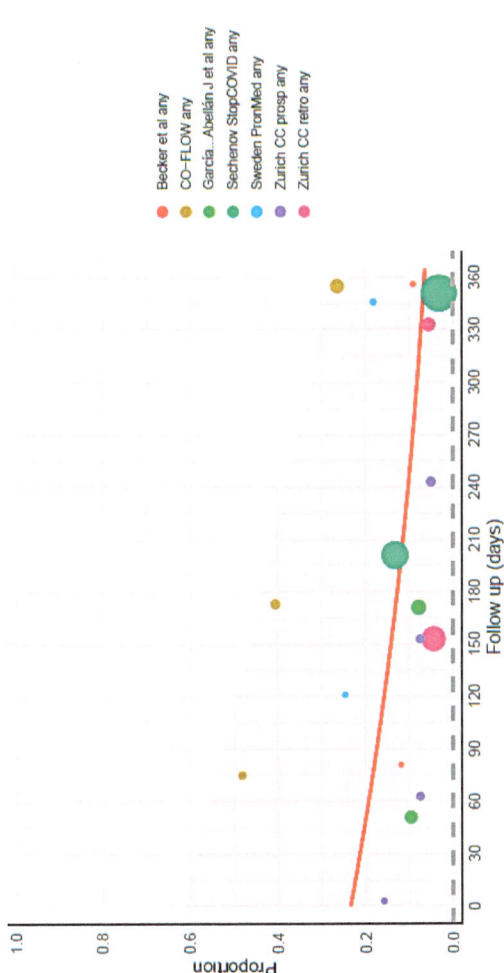

FIGURE 2-5 Duration of Long COVID among hospitalized COVID cases.[1]

[1] The speaker updated this figure after the presentation.

NOTE: Becker et al any = Becker et al., 2021; CO-FLOW any = Bek et al., 2021; Sechenov STOPCOVID any = Osmanov et al., 2022, and Munblit et al., 2021; Sweden PronMed any = Hultström et al., 2021, and Ekbom et al., 2021; Zurich CC prosp any = Prospective population in Puhan et al., 2021; Zurich CC retro any = Retrospective population in Puhan et al., 2021.

SOURCE: Hanson et al., 2022, Appendix 1, p. 42, in Theo Vos presentation, March 21, 2022.

TABLE 2-1 Probability of Ongoing Symptoms at 3, 6, and 12 Months after Acute COVID-19[a]

		Months Since End of Acute Episode		
Females		3 Mo	6 Mo	12 Mo
Community*	Children < 20	2.55%	1.26%	0.26%
Community	Adults ≥ 20	9.26%	4.88%	1.24%
Hospital	All Ages	33.64%	25.74%	13.94%
ICU	All Ages	51.49%	42.08%	25.37%
Males				
Community*	Children < 20	2.55%	1.26%	0.26%
Community	Adults ≥ 20	4.05%	2.05%	0.47%
Hospital	All Ages	20.84%	15.25%	7.73%
ICU	All Ages	35.56%	27.41%	15.00%
* Estimates for community cases among children are assumed the same for males and females				
All Surviving Cases				
Females		7.42%	4.05%	1.16%
Males		3.93%	2.10%	0.58%
Both Sexes		5.68%	3.07%	0.87%

[a] The speaker updated this table after the presentation.
SOURCE: Theo Vos presentation, March 21, 2022.

toward cases in which patients were hospitalized (20 percent), but the majority are still mild cases. About two-thirds of these cases are in females, and 70 percent are in people aged 20 to 64.

Vos shared the limitations of this research and the estimates. The data are sparse and heterogeneous, and relatively few studies are from low- and middle-income countries. Study protocols often lack follow-up to determine the "tail" of duration; only a few studies followed patients to the 12-month mark. Vos also said that symptom clusters used in the estimates may miss patients who have isolated symptoms. Lastly, these estimates do not include the heightened risk of diseases such as heart disease and stroke attributable to COVID-19 infection. Going forward, he said, important areas of research include the impact of Long COVID after 12 months and how the different variants may affect the risk and severity of Long COVID.

Vos concluded with a summary of the implications of the data:

- There is considerable risk of ongoing symptoms after acute SARS-COV2 infection.
- The risk is highest in young adults and females, which is very different from the pattern seen in severe acute COVID-19.
- The majority of Long COVID cases are in people of working age.
- Around 24 percent of those with Long COVID at 3 months continued to have symptoms at 12 months.[10]
- In the United States, in 2021, 720,000 people aged 20 and older reached the 1-year duration mark; in 2022, this number is estimated to be 520,000.
- Recovery for the vast majority of long COVID cases occurs within a year.
- Considerable support (e.g., rehabilitation, income) may be needed to help individuals with Long COVID transition back into the workforce when symptoms begin to wane.

IMPACT OF COVID-19 ON THE WORKFORCE

Rakesh Kochhar, senior researcher at Pew Research Center, gave workshop participants a broad overview of labor market trends for workers overall in the United States, as well as for the population of people with a disability. While labor market data do not identify people with Long COVID, he said, those who have Long COVID are likely represented in the population of people with a disability; unusual changes in the size of this population could signal the impact of the pandemic.

To begin, Kochhar discussed data comparing employment trends during the COVID-19 recession to trends during the Great Recession that began in 2008. There was a steep decline in employment in the spring of 2020, followed by a gradual return toward normal. During the Great Recession, in contrast, employment fell much more slowly and did not recover, even after 2 years. Similarly, said Kochhar, there was a sharp increase in unemployment at the beginning of the pandemic, with about 17 million people losing their jobs over the span of 2 months. Unemployment gradually declined but is still about 10 percent higher than in February 2020, he said. Unemployment during the Great Recession increased gradually and did not return to prerecession levels.

One key difference between the pandemic and the Great Recession, said Kochhar, is where job losses occurred (Figure 2-6). In the Great Reces-

---

[10] The speaker updated this figure after the presentation.

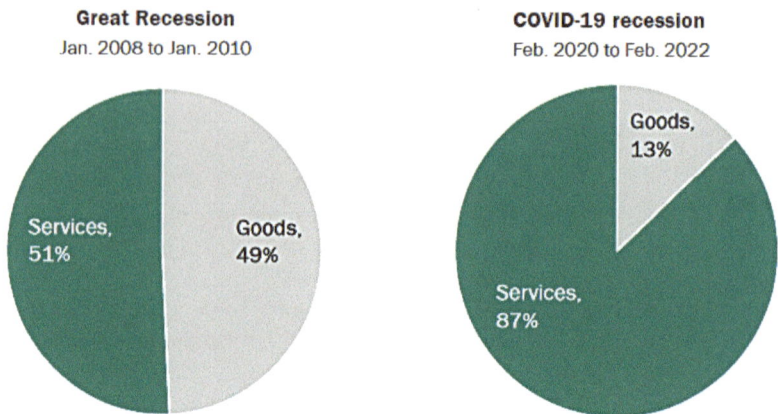

FIGURE 2-6 Share of a sector in total loss in employment.
SOURCE: Rakesh Kochhar presentation, March 21, 2022, based on data from the U.S. Bureau of Labor Statistics.

sion, about half of the job losses came from the goods sector, which includes manufacturing, construction, and mining. The goods sector only accounts for around 10 percent of overall employment in the United States, said Kochhar, and many of these lost jobs were middle wage jobs that are "still gone for good." In contrast, 87 percent of jobs lost during the pandemic came from the services sector; these were primarily low-wage workers who held jobs that did not offer the possibility of telecommuting. Women were hit harder by these initial losses, but parity has been restored in the longer run. Likewise, patterns of racial disparities persisted through the pandemic and the recovery. One "unusual" outlier, he said, was a spike in unemployment for Asian workers. These workers on average have high levels of education and low levels of unemployment, but many were in service jobs that were vulnerable during the pandemic (e.g., restaurants, dry cleaning). Comparing age groups, Kochhar said that the youngest workers were most affected; at one point, one in four workers aged 16 to 24 were unemployed. However, the ebb and flow of recovery has been similar for all age groups.

While the unemployment rate receives a great deal of attention, said Kochhar, the number of people who are not in the labor force at all is also an important indicator of labor market strength. There are around 100 million people currently not in the U.S. labor force, including those who are retired or otherwise not looking for or interested in work. The size of the labor force has not recovered to the extent that unemployment and employment have, said Kochhar; there are about four million more people not in the labor force compared to the beginning of the pandemic. Women have left the labor force at rates higher than men; Kochhar noted that women are more affected by school and daycare closures than men. About half of the workers who have left—2.4 million—were 55 and older. Some of these departures, he said, were likely workers retiring earlier than they had planned.

Next, Kochhar presented data from the U.S Bureau of Labor Statistics focused on the population of people with a disability in the United States.[11] About 31 million people aged 16 and over have a disability, which is around 700,000 people more than in 2019. This represents around 12 percent of the population. Hispanic adults account for a disproportionate share of the increase in the number of people with a disability, said Kochhar. Hispanics represent 17 percent of the adult population, and 12 percent of the population with a disability, yet they account for half of the recent increase in people with a disability. Another surprising development, he said, is that the number of young people (ages 16 to 24) with a disability increased by more than 200,000 people, accounting for close to one-third of the total increase in the population. Most people with a disability are not in the labor force and are not seeking work, said Kochhar. Out of 31 million, only around 7 million are in the labor force, working or looking for a job (Figure 2-7).

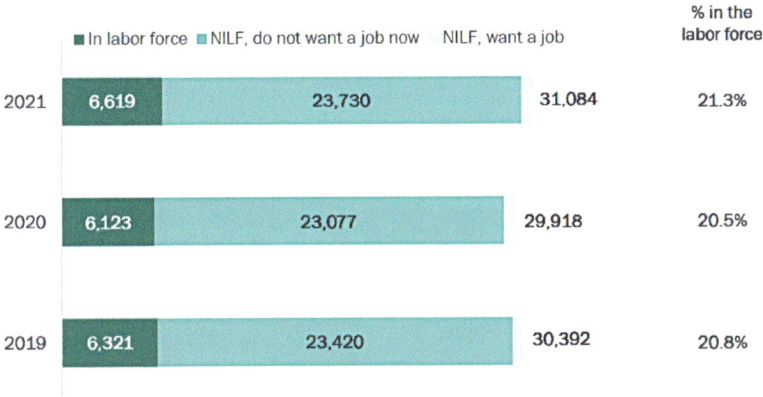

FIGURE 2-7 Number of people ages 16 and older with a disability, in thousands.
NOTE: NILF = not in the labor force.
SOURCE: Rakesh Kochhar presentation, March 21, 2022, based on data from the U.S. Bureau of Labor Statistics.

---

[11] People with a disability reported having at least one of the following conditions: deaf or serious difficulty hearing; blind or serious difficulty seeing; difficulty concentrating, remembering, or making decisions; difficulty walking or climbing stairs; difficulty dressing or bathing; and difficulty doing errands alone.

While the percentage of people with a disability who are employed is relatively low, employment has rebounded more quickly in this population compared to the population without disabilities (Figure 2-8). In the population of people without disabilities, the share employed is still several percentage points lower than in 2019, while in the population of people with disabilities, the share employed has nearly returned to prepandemic levels.

DISCUSSION

Following the presentations, Frontera moderated a question-and-answer session with panelists and workshop participants.

How should Long COVID be defined?

Vos replied that it is a matter of choice, noting that while his research uses the 3-month threshold suggested by WHO, the analyses can be conducted to make estimates at any period of time postinfection. Katz agreed that it is a matter of choice, saying that there are no strong data to support one definition versus another at this point in time.

Has the pandemic changed or accelerated any trends in the skills or abilities required for employment?

Kochhar said that he is not sure how things will play out in the next year or two, but that it is possible that the economy will be reshaped by changes in

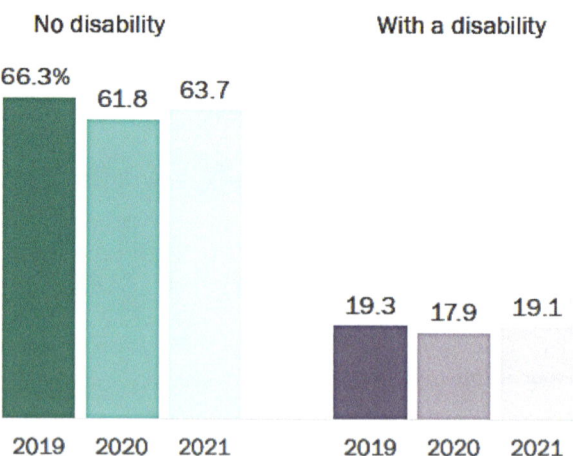

FIGURE 2-8 Percentage of population ages 16 and older that is employed.
SOURCE: Rakesh Kochhar presentation, March 21, 2022, based on data from the U.S. Bureau of Labor Statistics.

supply and demand. He noted that there was a shift toward a higher demand in the information technology sector during the pandemic.

Given that most Long COVID cases come from those with milder infections, what should clinicians be doing to follow up and investigate long-term symptoms in their patients?

"The most important thing for a clinician is to take this seriously," said Vos. The biggest hurdle for those with Long COVID is to be taken seriously by medical practitioners, he said, so there is a need for education for physicians so they know that Long COVID is a common occurrence, even in patients with mild infections. Katz agreed, noting that it is critical for primary care providers to recognize patients' symptoms and take them seriously.

Is there evidence about the length of time that it takes for post-COVID symptoms to return or relapse after they appear to have improved?

There are some data from symptom-tracking apps in the United Kingdom (Sudre et al., 2021), where people are asked to answer questions regularly about their symptoms, said Vos. These data give more of an idea of how symptoms change over time. Unfortunately, we do not have enough detailed data to quantify or model the waxing and waning of symptoms.

Is there any evidence about whether recurring COVID-19 infection increases the risk for Long COVID?

There is no evidence on this point, said Vos, but one might expect that additional contact with the virus may lead to additional risk or worsening of existing symptoms. Hanson added that future research will explore the effect of vaccination status on the risk of Long COVID.

In the model estimates, why was the decision made to assume that asymptomatic people do not develop Long COVID?

This decision, said Vos, was based on the fact that the small number of asymptomatic infections included in the cohort studies showed a very low proportion of cases that demonstrated the three symptom clusters, which are (1) fatigue, body pain, and depression/anxiety; (2) cognitive problems; and (3) ongoing respiratory problems. Further, it could not be determined whether the people were asymptomatic at the time of their test and remained asymptomatic, or whether they eventually developed symptoms. While the risk of Long COVID for asymptomatic individuals may not be zero, it appears to be significantly lower than for symptomatic individuals. Katz added that the RECOVER study is aiming to include a large proportion of asymptomatic individuals in the pediatric population, in order to better reflect the experience of this population. However, studying asymptomatic infection has many challenges, including how and when the infection is detected.

Given that many Long COVID symptoms are hard to diagnose or measure objectively (e.g., brain fog, fatigue), how should SSA evaluate health records to determine who meets the definition of disabled?

By the nature of these symptoms, said Vos, SSA will have to heavily rely on people's self-reporting. However, patient reports can be collected in a more systematic way by using identified measurement scales and symptom questions, and evaluation thresholds can be set on these tools.

Is there a way to track the level of infiltration of the virus in different organs or body systems, and would this information be useful, given what is known about the correlation between severity and long-term symptoms?

The usefulness of this information, said Vos, depends on the mechanism that leads to Long COVID. There are a number of hypotheses for the mechanism; some posit that Long COVID is caused by virus remaining in the body, while others believe it is an immune system overreaction to a past infection that leads to the symptoms. If it is caused by an immune system overreaction, said Vos, quantifying virus in the organs will not be of much help. Moreover, he said, the fact that so many cases of Long COVID occur in patients with mild infections suggests that there are other mechanisms at play. Katz added that the RECOVER study is collecting data to help answer these questions; there is an autopsy cohort in which tissues will be examined for viral persistence, and there will be a large biobank with blood samples that can be examined to explore hypotheses about mechanisms.

3

Postacute Sequelae of SARS-CoV-2 Infection and Implications for Recovery

Steven Deeks, professor of medicine in residence at the University of California, San Francisco, introduced the second session of the workshop. In this session, experts described the pathology and clinical presentation of symptoms caused by SARS-CoV-2, and they explored what is known about the mechanisms and long-term potential consequences of this disease in different body systems. Speakers discussed effects on the neurological, neuromuscular, neuropsychiatric, cardiovascular, pulmonary, and musculoskeletal systems, and explored the burden of pain and fatigue associated with Long COVID.

NEUROLOGICAL AND NEUROMUSCULAR SEQUELAE

There are acute, subacute, and chronic neurological complications of COVID-19, said Avi Nath, clinical director of the National Institute of Neurological Disorders and Stroke at the National Institutes of Health. In the acute phase, patients can suffer from anosmia, metabolic and hypoxic encephalopathy, strokes, and more rarely, viral encephalitis or sudden death caused by hypoventilation. Subacute sequelae are inflammatory syndromes and can include acute disseminated encephalomyelitis, acute necrotizing hemorrhagic encephalopathy, and limbic encephalitis; children can experience multisystem inflammatory syndrome (MIS-C). Chronic neurological complications fall under the umbrella of Long COVID.

When considering the pathology of neurological complications, said Nath, the first question is whether the virus actually invades the brain. While there is a potential route for SARS-CoV-2 to enter the brain through the olfactory pathway, Nath said that researchers have only very rarely detected virus in the brain; when it has been detected, it is in small amounts and is not accompanied by inflammation (Lee et al., 2021). However, the acute effect of COVID-19 on the brain can be severe. Patients may suffer from ischemic strokes, hemorrhage, and clots in venous sinuses. Autopsies of brain tissue have found fibrinogen leaking into the brain, as well as blood vessels that are almost completely occluded. These findings, said Nath, are uniquely associated with COVID-19. Tinnitus, dizziness, and vertigo are also common occurrences in patients with COVID-19 (Viola et al., 2021); the prevailing hypothesis is that these are caused by a vascular phenomenon affecting the small blood vessels in the ear.

Subacute conditions associated with COVID-19 include different types of neuroinflammation; Nath noted that many of these conditions are seen in other viral infections and thus are well characterized. These conditions may include acute disseminated encephalomyelitis, which is T cell mediated (Novi et al., 2020), and acute necrotizing hemorrhagic encephalopathy, which is cytokine mediated (Poyiadji et al., 2020). MIS-C in children is associated with acute symptoms including fever, dyspnea, rash, vomiting, and circulatory failure; longer-term symptoms include encephalopathy, dysarthria, dysphagia, and generalized flaccid weakness (Abdel-Mannan et al., 2020). Fortunately, said Nath, the neurological manifestations of MIS-C tend to respond to treatment with corticosteroids and intravenous immunoglobulin. In addition to inflammation in the brain, inflammation may also affect the peripheral nerves, including cranial nerves. Researchers have reported Miller Fisher syndrome, polyneuritis cranialis, ophthalmoparesis, and acute polyradiculitis in COVID-19 patients (Dias et al., 2021). These conditions also tend to respond well to corticosteroids, he said.

Most COVID-19 patients, said Nath, recover within 3 months (Whitaker et al., 2021). However, if they do not recover by this time, symptoms may not abate. Nath shared research from the National Health Service in the United Kingdom (Whitaker et al., 2021) that found that among those symptomatic at onset, 52 percent were symptomatic at 4 weeks, and 38 percent at 12 weeks. Those with more symptoms at the beginning tend to continue to have more symptoms, and women experience both more initial and lingering symptoms than men. Early manifestations of COVID-19, said Nath, may be useful for predicting what happens in the long term.

Some patients, however, fully recover from mild initial symptoms but then develop new symptoms days or weeks later. These symptoms tend to persist for extended periods of time. Nath mentioned that unpublished research data on a small cohort of these patients showed that nearly all reported cognitive dysfunction and fatigue, and smaller percentages reported palpitations, paresthesias, psychiatric issues, and dizziness. Long COVID symptoms, said

Nath, can be divided into four categories: exercise intolerance; cognition, mood, and sleep disorders; pain syndromes; and dysautonomia (Figure 3-1). Brain scans of patients experiencing Long COVID show morphological and metabolic changes in the brain, said Nath, including differences in amyloid proteins, decreased ratio of brain to total intracranial volume, and atrophy of olfactory tracks.

Nath ended with three main points:

- Direct invasion of the brain by SARS-CoV-2 is rare and does not explain the neurological complications.
- Neuroimmune dysfunction is driven by activation of innate immunity, immune exhaustion, and antibody-mediated phenomenon.
- Endothelial cell damage by immune complexes is the primary pathophysiological process in neuro-COVID.

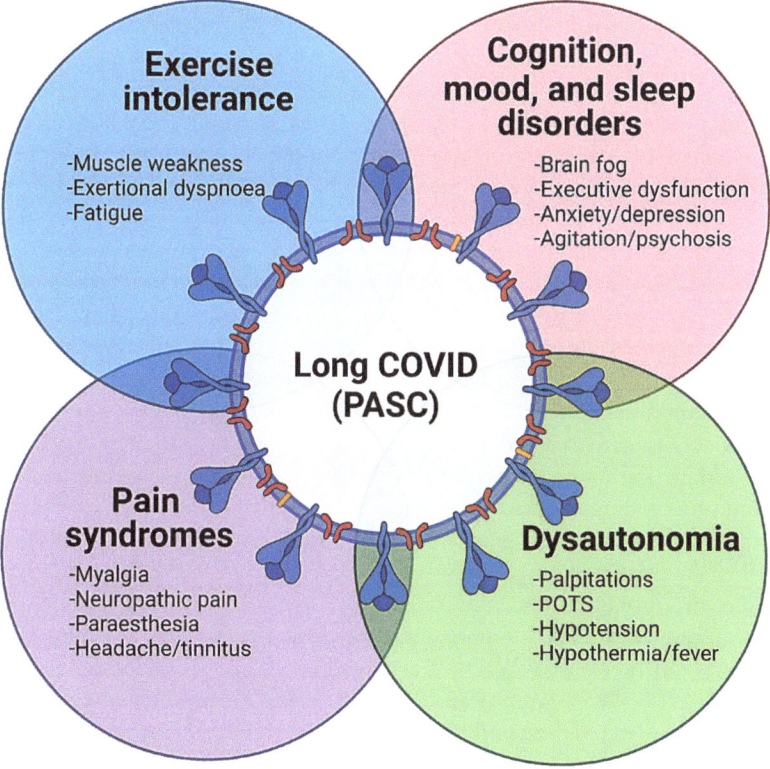

FIGURE 3-1 Long COVID symptoms.
NOTE: POTS = postural orthostatic tachycardia syndrome.
SOURCE: Balcom et al., 2021, p. 3581, in Avi Nath presentation, March 21, 2022.

NEUROPSYCHIATRIC SEQUELAE

Emily Troyer, director of the child and adolescent psychiatry track for the community psychiatry program at the University of California, San Diego, began by sharing a historical perspective from the influenza pandemic that began in 1918. Effects on physical and mental health were still reported many years later, said Troyer, which emphasizes that the full scope of neuropsychiatric sequelae following COVID-19 might not be known for years or even decades. Research on past coronavirus outbreaks—SARS (severe acute respiratory syndrome) and MERS (Middle East respiratory syndrome)—found that cognitive, mood, and trauma-related symptoms were common among survivors (Rogers et al., 2020). Further, she said, nearly a quarter of survivors had not returned to work 3 years postillness.

Psychiatric symptoms are commonly seen during the acute infection phase of COVID-19, as well as in the first 3 months following illness, said Troyer. Having a preexisting psychiatric disorder, particularly schizophrenia, has been associated with increased risk of COVID-19 infection, hospitalizations, and death. Longer-term psychiatric symptoms—those that occur more than 3 months after the acute phase of the illness—include sleep disturbance, depression, anxiety, and trauma-related symptoms. Psychosis is rare, said Troyer, but has been reported. Interestingly, she said, research does not show an association between the severity of the acute COVID-19 infection and the risk for depression or anxiety. In fact, some studies suggest that milder infection is actually associated with a greater risk for depression and anxiety. Troyer noted, however, that any of these studies have important limitations and further research is needed. One large retrospective study (Taquet et al., 2021) that used electronic health records to look at postinfection outcomes found that almost 24 percent of patients experienced a mood, anxiety, or psychotic disorder within the first 6 months, and that almost 9 percent of survivors experienced a disorder that was not present prior to COVID-19 infection. The study compared COVID-19 patients to survivors of influenza and other respiratory tract infections, and found that the risk of several psychiatric disorders was significantly greater following COVID-19 infection. These findings, said Troyer, point out the "scale of the issue facing us as we try to recover from the pandemic."

Troyer described the potential pathogenic mechanisms that create the association between COVID-19 and neuropsychiatric symptoms. In short, she said, it is "likely complex and multifactorial." One potential mechanism is inflammatory cytokines in the peripheral and central nervous systems shunting the brain's energy away from the production of neurotransmitters such as serotonin, dopamine, and norepinephrine, and toward the production of toxic metabolites such as quinolinic acid (Boldrini et al., 2021). Troyer noted that the lack of clinical or objective biomarkers for these processes makes it challenging to screen or diagnose patients at risk. Another potential mechanism for neuropsychiatric symptoms is the maternal immune activation hypothesis. This hypothesis suggests that individuals who are exposed to inflammation in utero—whether caused by infection, stress, or other causes—are at increased risk for neurodevelopmental disorders later in life. Going forward, said Troyer, it will be important to continue to try to understand how COVID-19 infection could affect individuals throughout their lives.

Neuropsychiatric sequelae in children following COVID-19 infection is much less well understood compared to adults, said Troyer. The good news, she said, is that the prevalence of Long COVID in children seems to be lower, with about one to five percent of youth who have had acute COVID experiencing Long COVID (Stephenson et al., 2021). The pandemic in general has negatively affected mental health among the youth, she added. Another interesting finding, she said, is that Danish teenagers who had a history of COVID-19 infection were more likely to miss school than teenagers who had not been infected, even though there were no reported differences in psychiatric or general health outcomes (Kikkenborg Berg et al., 2022). This finding, said Troyer, suggests a possible mismatch between reported mental health impairment and actual functional impairment in children.

Troyer summarized her main points:

- COVID-19 infection is associated with a risk for exacerbation of and new-onset psychiatric disorders, including mood, anxiety, and trauma-related disorders, as well as sleep disturbances.
- Nearly all studies to date have been conducted in adult samples, and findings may not be generalizable to other stages of human development.
- Longer-term outcomes, pathogenic mechanisms, biomarkers, and effective treatments for post-COVID-19 psychiatric disorders remain to be elucidated.
- Disentangling effects of COVID-19 infection versus pandemic-related stress will be difficult, as both may contribute to long-term sequelae via neuroimmune mechanisms.
- The scale of the pandemic will require that brain and mental health be integral components of research and clinical and social service planning in the coming years.

CARDIOVASCULAR SEQUELAE AND AUTONOMIC SYNDROME

Survey data show that a significant proportion of patients with PASC report symptoms of autonomic dysfunction,[1] said Peter Novak, director of the Autonomic Laboratory at Brigham and Women's Hospital. To characterize and understand the autonomic symptoms associated with PASC, Novak and his colleagues designed a retrospective study that enrolled patients with PASC who were experiencing fatigue and brain fog (Novak et al., 2022). The protocol for evaluating patients consisted of cerebrovascular, respiratory, autonomic, and small fiber assessment, as well as testing for markers of low-grade inflammation. The first cohort of patients were nine white women, all of whom had mild COVID-19 and none of whom were vaccinated. These patients were age and sex matched with 10 women who had postural orthostatic tachycardia syndrome (POTS) and 15 healthy controls.[2] Novak noted that the POTS controls were used because there is a great deal of overlap in terms of presentation and clinical findings between patients with POTS and those with PASC.

Novak described the study findings. Small fiber neuropathy (damage of the nerves) was found in 89 percent of patients with PASC, 60 percent of patients with POTS, and none of the healthy controls. Cerebrovascular dysregulation was found in all PASC patients; the pattern of decrease in cerebral blood flow velocity while in a tilted position was similar between POTS and PASC patients. In addition, said Novak, dysautonomia in at least one domain was found in all of the PASC and POTS patients and in none of the healthy controls.[3] Respiratory dysregulation occurred in 100 percent of PASC patients, in 75 percent of POTS patents, and in none of the healthy controls. Elevated inflammatory markers were found in 67 percent of PASC patients and 70 percent of POTS patients, but the markers were heterogeneous and there was no typical pattern.

In concluding, Novak described the implications of this research:

---

[1] The autonomic nervous system is a control system that acts largely unconsciously and regulates bodily functions, such as the heart rate, digestion, respiratory rate, pupillary response, urination, and sexual arousal.

[2] POTS is an autonomic nervous system disorder that creates an abnormal increase in heart rate that occurs after sitting up or standing. The various symptoms of POTS, including dizziness and fainting, can range from mild to disabling.

[3] Dysautonomia refers to medical conditions caused by problems with the autonomic nervous system. These disorders can be mild to debilitating, and usually involve abnormal symptoms in many organ systems, including cardiac, gastrointestinal, neurological, and pulmonary, and others.

- PASC is associated with multisystem dysfunction affecting the cerebrovascular, autonomic, peripheral, respiratory, and inflammatory systems; this is most likely caused by low-grade inflammation that is either systemic or targets the vascular system.
- A number of clinical manifestations are correlated with system dysfunction, including pain and sensory disturbances (neuropathy); orthostatic intolerance, fatigue, and brain fog (cerebrovascular dysregulation); dyspnea and increased fatigue (respiratory dysregulation); and fatigue, exercise intolerance, dry mouth, and urinary and GI symptoms (dysautonomia). Several studies have confirmed these findings.
- The severity of the symptoms experienced by PASC patients is similar to the severity of symptoms experienced by patients with other disabling conditions, including POTS, chronic fatigue syndrome, and small fiber neuropathy.

PULMONARY SEQUELAE

Breathlessness is a common symptom of COVID-19, but it is a complex and multifactorial symptom, said Ann Marie Parker, intensivist and assistant professor of pulmonary and critical care medicine at the Johns Hopkins School of Medicine. Recent data (Montani et al., 2022) show that breathlessness is the most common respiratory symptom reported at 12 months with between 5 to 81 percent of previously hospitalized patients experiencing breathlessness, and around 14 percent of nonhospitalized patients. Breathlessness is not closely associated with the initial severity of COVID-19, said Parker; patients with mild or severe initial illness can have long-lasting breathlessness. Cough is also commonly reported, with between 2 and 42 percent of PASC patients experiencing cough (Montani et al., 2022). Both breathlessness and cough are associated with worse quality of life, said Parker.

Parker gave an overview of the incidence and prevalence of post-COVID-19 respiratory sequelae, noting that most evidence comes from China and Europe because they are ahead of the United States in the timeline of the pandemic. One study (Huang et al., 2021a) found that among patients who were hospitalized but largely not in the ICU, about 75 percent had one symptom at 6 months, and about 25 percent had breathlessness. The most common abnormality in pulmonary function testing was a decrease in oxygen diffusing capacity, and some patients had abnormal physical function, as demonstrated by a low score on the 6-minute walk test. Patients who had required respiratory support during hospitalization were more likely to report breathlessness and decreased mobility at 6 months, she said. A follow-up study (Huang et al., 2021b) observed a subset of these patients at 12 months. About half reported one symptom, and about 30 percent reported breathlessness at 1 year. Pulmonary function and physical function tests did not show improvement between 6 months and 12 months. However, she said, the proportion of patients with restrictive lung disease decreased, from about 40 percent at 6 months to about 30 percent at 12 months.

Another study (Wu et al., 2021) prospectively followed 83 patients who were hospitalized with severe COVID-19 but who did not receive steroids or other medications that are now used. Patients who had preexisting comorbidities were excluded to isolate the pulmonary complications of COVID-19 itself. The most common symptom at 3, 6, and 12 months was mild to moderate decrease in oxygen diffusing capacity,[4] which generally improved over time. Physical function as measured by the 6-minute walk test and abnormalities on chest imaging similarly improved over time. However, said Parker, a quarter of patients still had abnormal chest imaging at 12 months, and in these patients the need for respiratory support or having a long hospital stay were associated with this outcome. A third of patients continued to have a decrease in oxygen diffusing capacity at 12 months; females were more likely than males to experience this complication (Wu et al., 2021).

These studies, Parker observed, demonstrate that pulmonary complications after COVID-19 infection tend to be mild to moderate and tend to improve over time without intervention. Parker described the reasons patients might report a perception of breathlessness following an acute COVID-19 infection; one reason, for example, is asthma. Parker indicated there is no robust evidence confirming the hypothesis that people with asthma might be susceptible to more severe COVID-19. A few studies have looked at the long-term outcomes of patients with asthma after a COVID-19 infection, said Parker. One study (Philip et al., 2022) of 471 patients with asthma and self-reported COVID-19 infection found that about half reported experiencing Long COVID. A greater percentage of those with Long COVID reported worsened breathing, an increase in rescue inhaler use, and worsened asthma management. In addition to asthma, other factors that could contribute to a perception of breathlessness, said Parker, include hyperventilation, peripheral deconditioning, respiratory or diaphragmatic weakness, interstitial lung disease, pulmonary embolism, cardiovascular complications, POTS, and chronic fatigue syndrome. Evaluation of patients with respiratory complications from COVID-19 can include chest imaging, pulmonary function tests, CT scans, walk tests, and echocardiogram (George et al., 2020). Parker noted that

---

[4] Diffusing capacity is a measure of how well oxygen and carbon dioxide are transferred (diffused) between the lungs and the blood and can be a useful test in the diagnosis and treatment monitoring of lung diseases.

because there are no COVID-19-specific interventions in the post-COVID care setting, referring patients to subspecialists is appropriate.

Parker summarized three main points:

- Breathlessness and cough are common following acute COVID-19 infections; they are complex and multifactorial symptoms.
- Few COVID-19-specific therapeutic options exist, so treatments are based on what is known about related conditions (e.g., asthma).
- Research priorities include investigations of the natural history of the disease; risk factors (patient specific, acute phase, and recovery); therapeutic interventions; and long-term patient-centered outcomes.

MUSCULOSKELETAL, FATIGUE, AND PAIN SEQUELAE

Anthony Komaroff, professor of medicine at Harvard Medical School and senior physician at Brigham and Women's Hospital, gave participants an overview of what is known about musculoskeletal symptoms, fatigue, postexertional malaise, and pain in people with Long COVID. The incidence of Long COVID, and the associated sequelae, is difficult to determine because studies have used a variety of designs and definitions, he said. For example, some studies require COVID-19 to be diagnosed by a lab test, while others accept self-report; some use electronic health records to track symptoms, while others survey patients about their symptoms. However, some evidence can be gleaned from the existing studies, said Komaroff.

One systematic review of 57 studies (Groff et al., 2021) found frequent persistent symptoms in patients 6 months after a COVID-19 infection, including fatigue, pain, postexertion malaise, and loss of mobility and function. Komaroff explained that postexertional malaise is a cardinal symptom of myalgic encephalomyelitis/chronic fatigue syndrome (ME/CFS); it is defined as prolonged exacerbation of patient's baseline symptoms after physical, cognitive, or orthostatic exertion or stress (IOM, 2015). The exacerbation of symptoms may be delayed relative to the trigger, he said; for example, in people with ME/CFS, physical exertion does not produce the symptoms until 12 to 48 hours after exertion. A study that conducted cardiopulmonary exercise testing (Singh et al., 2022) found that while peak cardiac index did not differ between patients with Long COVID and healthy controls, the Long COVID patients had significantly lower levels of peak VO2 and systematic oxygen extraction. This suggests, said Komaroff, an underlying physiologic abnormality that is correlated with and could explain some of the postexertional malaise found in Long COVID patients.

Another study (Beauchamp et al., 2022) found that people with probable or confirmed acute COVID-19 infections were more likely to experience functional impairment than those without a history of COVID-19 infections. Over the 9-month study period, COVID-19 patients were about twice as likely to have a reduced ability to engage in normal household activities, reduced physical activity, and difficulty standing from a sitting position. Fatigue following an infection is not unique to COVID-19, said Komaroff. Similar symptoms have been found in patients infected with viral, bacterial, and protozoal infections ranging from Ebola to Lyme disease to enteroviruses.

A number of similarities exist between Long COVID and ME/CFS, said Komaroff, with similarities both in symptoms and in pathophysiology. Studies that examined whether and to what extent Long COVID patients resembled patients with ME/CFS found that 6 to 9 months after acute COVID-19, between 13 and 25 percent of patients met the diagnostic criteria for ME/CFS (González-Hermosillo et al., 2021; Mirfazeli et al., 2022; Townsend et al., 2020). Similarities between Long COVID and ME/CFS include:

- Dysautonomia/brainstem dysfunction
- Autoantibodies, many to neural targets
- Decreased generation of ATP[5]
- General hypometabolic state, including in brain
- Gut microbiome dysbiosis
- Endothelial dysfunction and coagulopathy
- Small fiber neuropathy
- Cognitive deficits
- Neuroinflammation

Researchers are exploring a number of potential biological triggers for this wide range of pathophysiology, said Komaroff, including inflammation caused by injury and repair in multiple organs; persistent reservoirs of the virus in the body that generate a chronic immune response; integration of the viral genome into the host genome; reactivation of neurotropic pathogens; mitochondrial dysfunction; and chronic inflammation and autoimmunity caused by gut dysbiosis.

To summarize, Komaroff stated the following points:

- Musculoskeletal disease and symptoms, fatigue, postexertional malaise, and pain can often persist for at least 6 months following acute COVID-19.
- Functional impairment, often attributed to these symptoms, is common.

---

[5] ATP stands for adenosine triphosphate, a molecule that provides energy to drive many processes in living cells.

- Long COVID patients have similar symptoms to people with ME/CFS and other postinfectious syndromes.
- Long COVID and ME/CFS appear to have similar underlying pathophysiology.

DISCUSSION

Deeks moderated a question-and-answer session between workshop participants and the panelists.

Given that the pandemic had a huge impact on everyone's mental health, how do we distinguish between mental health issues that are potentially related to Long COVID and general mental health issues?

"We will never have a nonpandemic exposed control group," said Troyer, which makes it very difficult to measure and disentangle mental health issues that are related to COVID-19 infection. There is an increased prevalence of a lot of different mental health conditions, she said, but specific conditions are being observed in Long COVID patients, including cognitive dysfunction and fatigue. While idiopathic psychiatric conditions can also cause dysfunction and fatigue, the mechanisms are likely different for Long COVID patients. Interestingly, she continued, there is evidence that standard treatments for mental health conditions, such as selective serotonin reuptake inhibitors (SSRIs), may affect COVID-19 infection and severity. This creates a possibility for a better understanding of how standard psychiatric treatments affect other body systems, and how COVID-19 treatments (e.g., anti-inflammatory agents) may affect psychiatric outcomes. This relationship, said Troyer, may start to "break down some of the barriers between psychiatric and medical illness."

What are the differences and similarities between Long COVID and POTS? Are POTS treatments working in Long COVID patients?

The traditional presentation of POTS, said Novak, is a young female who develops orthostatic intolerance and tachycardia palpitation after an infection, usually a viral infection. There are a lot of similarities between Long COVID and POTS; for example, the decrease in orthostatic blood flow velocity is similar in patients, although the mechanisms may be different. Reduced orthostatic cerebral blood flow velocity can result in cerebral hypoperfusion that can be linked to brain fog and fatigue. Immunomodulatory treatments used for some patients with POTS may be effective for Long COVID, such as intravenous immunoglobulin and steroids. Novak said that diagnosing these syndromes can be challenging, and that it typically requires finding a correlation between objective evidence and the symptoms that the patient reports.

What is the potential relationship, if any, between post-ICU syndrome and Long COVID?

Prior to COVID-19, patients who were in the ICU with acute respiratory distress syndrome experienced functional impairment after their ICU stay that seemed to be driven by neuromuscular and psychiatric impairments, rather than pulmonary complications, said Parker. Patients who have been in the ICU have high rates of anxiety, depression, posttraumatic stress disorder (PTSD), and cognitive impairment, she said, and decline in physical function is extremely common. Parker said that half of ICU patients have not returned to work 1 year after their stay in the ICU. Even if the specific effects of the SARS-CoV-2 virus could be isolated, Parker said we could anticipate that COVID-19 would further exacerbate recovery from critical illness. For example, patients in the ICU during the pandemic may not have access to early rehabilitation or may not be able to have visitors because of infection and prevention control measures. These differences could further impair physical and cognitive recovery, as well as exacerbate anxiety, depression, and PTSD symptoms. "The truth is, we don't know" how post-ICU syndrome and Long COVID may be related, said Parker, and it will take rigorous prospective cohort studies to tease out the relationship.

What diagnostic tests are used in the clinic to help diagnose Long COVID, and to what extent are these tests able to assess patient functioning or predict their functioning in the future?

What is important to keep in mind, said Parker, is that many patients with Long COVID are not able to do the things they need and want to do on a regular basis. Identifying the functional impairment and considering potential contributors are first and foremost. For some patients, she said the issue could be neuromuscular weakness, for others it could be pulmonary issues, and others may have symptoms that are related to ME/CFS. While CT scans, echocardiograms, or other such tools are important for investigating dysfunction, more weight placed on the findings of tests that measure function (e.g., pulmonary function tests) is needed. She noted that radiological improvement and functional improvement may not always go hand in hand. The starting point for assessment, she said, should be the patient's functional impairment, rather than the results of clinical tests.

Komaroff identified some of the functional tests used in the assessment of Long COVID patients, including the 10-minute NASA Lean Test (Lee et al., 2020), which demonstrates similarly abnormal orthostatic function in patients with ME/CFS and Long COVID. The most important kind of tests, he said, are those that assess the stamina of people both physically and cognitively on repetitive challenges, because this deficit is commonly seen in people with ME/CFS and Long COVID.

In terms of using tests to predict longer-term outcomes, said Novak, we can possibly extrapolate from other conditions. For example, if someone has postviral small fiber neuropathy, it will likely take longer than 6 months to recover.

Why do females seem to be disproportionately affected by Long COVID?

Females are disproportionately affected by many autoimmune disorders, said Komaroff, and, with animal models for autoimmune diseases, if you give the males female hormones, they become more affected by these disorders. He said that there is "no doubt" in his mind that this difference is caused by hormones, but the mechanism by which sex hormones affect the expression of autoimmunity is unclear. Komaroff shared his hypothesis that female hormones increase the production and levels of autoantibodies, which explains some of the pathology. Troyer said there are also sex disparities in psychiatric disorders, with depression and anxiety more common in women, and autism and schizophrenia more common in men. One hypothesis is that it is related to inflammation, because there are hormone receptors for most of the inflammatory cytokines. Nath observed that there are multiple mechanisms by which symptoms and conditions can be affected, and the important thing is to figure out the underlying phenomenon and target that.

How do race and ethnicity factor into the risk for, and treatment of, Long COVID?

There is no doubt, said Nath, that African Americans and Hispanics have an increased risk of acquiring COVID-19 because of socioeconomic factors related to neighborhood or occupation, for example. In health care, the search for a genetic basis for patient differences is important, but so is an understanding of socioeconomic factors. Troyer said that issues of access are critical as well. For example, if a Long COVID patient needs to document her condition for the purposes of an SSA disability application, she may need to visit specialists for repeated testing over time. Accessing this care may be more difficult for low-income people or people of certain racial and ethnic groups. When determining whether and how to incorporate Long COVID into SSA disability programs, it is critical that disparities are not exacerbated, said Troyer.

4

Patient and Caregiver Perspectives on Living with Long COVID

This session, said Mansoor Malik, clinical professor of psychiatry at Johns Hopkins University, brings together individuals "trying to manage their lives living with a variety of conditions and symptoms that present challenges in every aspect of their lives." Their perspectives as a patient or caregiver, said Malik, uniquely reflects the range of outcomes and experiences following COVID-19 infection. The individuals first shared their stories via prerecorded video, then Malik moderated a panel discussion.

PATIENT STORIES

Angela Meriquez Vázquez

Vázquez is a disabled former athlete, a Long COVID patient, and the president of Body Politic, a grassroots patient-led organization for Long COVID advocacy. Before getting COVID-19, said Vázquez, she was a runner for nearly 2 decades. The morning of the day she started feeling sick with COVID-19, she went for a run, but she has not run since. For Vázquez, COVID-19 started as a mild illness that progressed over weeks with an "increasingly scary set of symptoms," including blood clots, ministrokes, brain swelling, seizures, heart palpitations, shortness of breath, confusion, numbness that progressed to an inability to walk for several days, and anaphylaxis. Now with Long COVID, Vázquez has several chronic conditions, including a mild form of ME/CFS. Because of this condition, if Vázquez pushes herself past a dynamic threshold, she will experience a relapse of symptoms like insomnia, brain fog, sleep apnea, and migraines. Vázquez said that she has developed a "strict pacing regimen" that allows her to work from home more than full time, but she does not do much else. "I don't socialize or enjoy my old hobbies, and I don't leave my home, especially now that I'm considered high risk," she said. Vázquez said that she is on the "mild end of the spectrum" of disability among Long COVID patients, and that she is lucky to have had access to patient support. She was guided to the right specialists who were "armed with research" on conditions such as POTS and ME/CFS, and potential treatments.

"We are living through what is likely to be the largest mass disabling event in modern history," said Vázquez, and noted that the virus has disproportionately affected communities of color. There are likely millions of Long COVID patients who remain unidentified and unsupported, she said, and there is an "imperative for large-scale change."

Treva Marie Taylor

Taylor was working as assistant director of hospitals for New York City Health and Hospitals Corporation when she contracted COVID-19 and was in the ICU at NYU Langone Health for 6 weeks. Her lungs collapsed, her organs failed, and she experienced hemorrhaging, blood clots, emphysema, and brain damage. "This disease is devastating," she said, and it will "cripple you from the head of you to the bottom of you in everything that you do." Because of COVID-19, she was without income for 6 months; she was fortunate to have family that could help. A little more than a year after her acute COVID-19 infection, she deals with intense fatigue and difficulty thinking, requires oxygen supplementation, and her "life consists" of going to therapy and doctor's appointments multiple times per week. In order to run an errand or simply go outside, she has to figure out how to bring her oxygen tanks and a portable backup, and often needs someone with her because of her fatigue. Despite her challenges, Taylor said she is hopeful that she will get better and stronger.

Juan Lewis

Lewis contracted COVID-19 in April 2020 while on a work assignment in Germany. He was hospitalized in the Netherlands, including a long stay in the ICU, then underwent rehab in the Netherlands before relocation to San Antonio, Texas. Lewis said that in April of 2020 he was "fighting for my life" and since September of 2020 he has been "fighting for my quality of life." Before COVID-19, he said, he exercised every day, had a perfect attendance record at work, received merit promotions, and was always at the top of his class. The last time he was in a hospital was 1965. After COVID-19, he is challenged with multiple symptoms, including congestive heart failure, reduced lung capacity, balance issues, brain fog, lack of smell, memory issues, headache, and gastrointestinal issues. One of Lewis' biggest challenges has been chronic fatigue. Fatigue doesn't "fit my personality," he said, and it has caused issues with anxiety and depression. The financial burdens have also been a challenge, as his wife had to quit her job to stay home and take care of him.

People with Long COVID may have difficulty processing instructions or remembering what was said, said Lewis, and he encouraged medical professionals and others to ensure patients fully understand. He said that he has spent a lot of money "trying to find the magic bullet" to cure his Long COVID and appreciates the workshop's focus on the issue. Lewis said that one of his recovery goals was to run a 5K race, but a medical professional had told him it would never be possible. He reported that over the weekend he was able to complete the race.

Lucas and Karin Denault

Lucas Denault contracted COVID-19 in January of 2021, as a 15-year-old student. His entire family had COVID-19, said his mother, Karin Denault, and they considered themselves "lucky and blessed" because they were all either asymptomatic or had very mild symptoms. Lucas was able to do his homework, work out, go outside to play, and attend remote school. However, about 6 weeks after exposure to COVID-19, he had a "massive decline in exercise tolerance." Lucas said that he went from a "packed life" full of school and athletics and social events to a life of remote school and lacking the energy to even talk to friends. By the end of April, the family sought help at a Long COVID clinic. The clinic diagnosed Lucas with POTS; his main symptoms are fatigue, nausea, dizziness, headaches, brain fog, exercise intolerance, and heat intolerance. One of the biggest challenges, he said, is "just feeling sick all the time." He said he feels like he "can't escape" the feeling of being sick, and it really hinders his quality of life.

Almost a year after Lucas' diagnosis with POTS, said his mother, he can attend school most of the time although there are days and weeks that he has to stay home. It is a "struggle to balance" his physical, emotional, cognitive, and social capabilities and needs every day. It is "like a guessing game," said Lucas, to figure out what classes and activities he is able to take on for the day, knowing that if he pushes himself too much it can set him back weeks. Karin said that Long COVID has been debilitating for Lucas and has also been challenging for his family, friends, and teachers. It is difficult because he looks like a "normal teenage boy" who should be trying his absolute best at school and sports, but his "absolute best looks a little different now" because of Long COVID. Lucas conveyed that he wants to help people with Long COVID get the help they need, and to help others understand how Long COVID and POTS can affect people no matter what they look like on the outside. His mother said that they are hoping to find help and relief so that he can get his future "back on track."

DISCUSSION

These stories, said Malik, have demonstrated the suffering but also the hope and courage of individuals with Long COVID. Malik asked the speakers questions, some of which came from workshop participants.

Can you describe some of the frustrations you dealt with when experiencing symptoms without a clear cause or simple diagnostic test? How did you and your health care providers navigate the lack of information about Long COVID effects? Did you ever feel your providers were working against you rather than with you, and if so, how was that resolved?

Vázquez began by saying that "early on in the pandemic, I was met with nothing but resistance from medical providers." When she began experiencing symptoms of COVID-19, her primary care provider told her not to come in for a test because "if you don't have COVID-19, you'll certainly get it" at the doctor's office. The lack of a confirmatory positive test has "haunted" Vázquez ever since, and being denied a test "set the stage" for every subsequent interaction she had with a medical provider. When she began experiencing cardiovascular symptoms and other Long COVID complications, medical professionals all referred to the lack of a positive test and told her she was just "pandemic anxious." Vázquez was discharged several times from the ER, with her stroke-like symptoms being interpreted as a psychiatric crisis. In these early days, Vázquez said she was "saved" by the emotional and tactical support of Long COVID patients and other chronically ill and disabled patients. About 3 months into her Long COVID symptoms, Vázquez changed to a new primary provider who immediately recognized her symptoms as potentially related to POTS and Mast Cell Activation Syndrome (MCAS). However, the lack of a positive test has continued to be a barrier; she has been denied access to every Long COVID clinic in Los Angeles.

Karin Denault said that accessing good health care for Lucas was really tough in the beginning. They saw multiple specialists, one of whom asked Lucas to run on a treadmill after being told that Lucas could barely get out of bed or attend school. Lucas said he was "excited" to run after not exercising in 2 months, but that afterward he felt very nauseous. The specialist said, "Everything looks fine," while Lucas thought, "I definitely don't feel fine." This experience of being brushed off, said Lucas, shows the lack of education and information available to providers. Karin said it took Lucas about 30 minutes to walk out of the specialist's office, and that no one came to check on them. Karin called the Kennedy Krieger Institute, distraught, and managed to get an appointment for the next day. She said that the worst part of their experience were feelings of hopelessness in the beginning.

How well do standard functional tests (e.g., 6-minute walk test, strength testing, IQ testing) capture your symptoms? How do you describe harder-to-measure symptoms to your caregivers?

Lewis said that it can be difficult to capture Long COVID symptoms because they come and go, and various symptoms appear at different times. For example, when he saw a cardiologist, his heart looked fine, but a pulmonologist noticed that his resting heart rate was dangerously low. Lewis said that although his doctor has been a "godsend," some doctors "make you feel real bad and make you feel like you're not sick" when symptoms cannot be readily explained. Taylor said that her symptoms also tend to come and go, which makes them difficult to capture in a standard test. For example, she said she might do great on the treadmill one day but the next day she can barely do anything, or she uses up all her energy in a test and then feels terrible the rest of the day.

Vázquez said that her postexertional symptom exacerbation is very difficult to capture because it happens after the testing occurs. For example, she said she could easily run a mile in order to check her cardiovascular and pulmonary function, but after the test she would experience "crushing fatigue, muscular pain, joint pain, migraines, insomnia, sleep apnea, and a whole host of other symptoms" over the next 24 to 48 hours. This is a piece that is often not discussed in the moment of being tested or talking with a provider about functionality, she said, and it is important to think about when considering someone's ability to work. Vázquez said that although she continued to work during her worst days, she was crashing every night, unable to do housework, and living in pain. Postexertional symptom exacerbation is a key symptom of both ME/CFS and Long COVID, she said, and we need to improve ways to assess its impact on patients' lives.

The uncertainty and unpredictability of Long COVID symptoms seem to be one of the hardest aspects. How have you had to change your functioning and daily life to account for that variability? How do you cope with the pressure to resume normal activities?

Karin Denault said that while medical professionals are getting better about acknowledging Long COVID, many lay people still do not understand it. She said that people joke that Lucas is just being "lazy" or does not want to go to school, when in fact he is "the most motivated person I know." Lewis agreed, saying that even his wife initially did not understand how sick he felt because he looked perfectly normal. Lewis made an analogy to a cell phone that did not get fully charged but can make one phone call; like the phone, he can sometimes function normally but afterward he will need to recharge again. Lucas said that his daily life has been "completely flipped upside down" because of the unpredictability and uncertainty of his symptoms. He had big plans for his junior year of high school but has found it difficult to do much more than schoolwork. Even doing an hour of schoolwork can give him brain fog, headache, and nausea, so he takes a break to try to control his symptoms so he can get back to work because "life moves on." Lucas said that his current approach to pushing through is not sustainable, and that he hits a regression every 3 months or so where everything catches up with him. The uncertainty is difficult, added his mother, because some days he wakes up and feels like he can take on the day but by midmorning he is ready to come home due to brain fog, dizziness, and nausea.

Vázquez agreed that the uncertainty and variability is incredibly hard, and it makes it difficult to know if she is seeing any improvement overall. For example, she said, 2 weeks ago she was feeling better and thought she might be in remission. However, after a stressful week, she was trying to fill out a form and had a "mental crash" to the extent that she was misspelling her own name and was uncertain if she was holding the pencil correctly. Looking back, Vázquez said that her body had been sending her signals to slow down, but that it can be difficult to heed these calls until her body shuts itself down.

Did you receive support from SSA, Medicaid, or employers' worker compensation support? If not, what were the barriers to getting support, and what support did you need?

Lewis has received support from the worker's compensation program, and it has been "a lot of paperwork." He said they are "constantly sending documentation" to fill out, and they have required him to seek second opinions far from his home. The paperwork and other requirements are challenging, he said, and they often "play ping pong" sending papers back and forth until they are accepted. He said that people often give instructions too quickly and encouraged programs, clinicians, and others who work with patients with Long COVID to be patient and to understand that their mental capacity may be challenged.

Taylor agreed that the red tape and paperwork involved with her city benefits are enormously challenging. For over 30 years, Taylor worked in the health care field, handling paperwork, managing difficult cases, and solving problems. Now she struggles to understand and fill out paperwork, and people question her lack of ability because she looks and sounds fine to them. Taylor said she would "love for someone to walk with me for 1 day just to see what it's like to get through a day."

From a health system perspective, what kind of information, actions, or policies are needed to help people with Long COVID recover?

One of the things that we have heard a lot is the lack of clinical education for doctors, said Vázquez. Because we are living through a mass disabling event, she said, we cannot continue to rely on specialists to provide ongoing clinical care to Long COVID patients. Even before the pandemic, there was a lack of capacity to treat complex and poorly understood conditions like POTS, mast cell activation syndrome (MCAS), and ME/CFS; now the population of these patients has "simply exploded." A massive education effort of primary care and pediatric clinicians is needed, said Vázquez, so that they can serve as the first line of screening and initial assessment. This will require the health care system to "get much more comfortable" with understanding and diagnosing these conditions, she said, emphasizing that even when clinical diagnostic criteria are in place, some patients on the margins will need and deserve care. Care and benefits should not be denied or delayed to this growing population just because the necessary investments before the pandemic to define and treat many of these conditions had not been in place. Malik added that even if few treatments are available for these conditions, patients need validation and care for their symptoms from doctors and caregivers.

What has been the effect of COVID-19 and Long COVID on your finances, your personal relationships, and your caregiver networks?

Taylor said she went without income for 6 months, which required her to drain her savings and to rely on help from her family, friends, and strangers. She now receives Social Security benefits, but she is still relying on her savings and her pension to survive. Lewis and his wife had to sell their home and buy a single-story home because of his inability to walk up and down stairs repeatedly. His symptoms have also affected his relationship with his new granddaughter; he said he avoids picking her up and holding her because he is afraid he will get dizzy and fall over. Karin Denault said that Lucas is fortunate because both of his parents were able to continue to work and had savings available to pay his medical bills.

For Vázquez, the biggest effect of Long COVID was in the workplace. She had just started a new job when she got sick, and she did not feel like she could take time off of work or reveal her struggles to her employer. She said she was not certain if she could even get accommodations because at the time, she was being told her symptoms were all in her head. Vázquez hid her disabilities and her condition from her employer for many months, for fear of not being believed or of losing her job. She noted that her employer-based health insurance is critical to her care, and that it feels like she is working to get health care, and that this health care is the only thing that allows her to work.

5

Long-Term Impairments and Functional Limitations Related to Long COVID

Laura Malone, pediatric neurologist and codirector of the Pediatric Post COVID-19 Rehabilitation Clinic at the Kennedy Krieger Institute, introduced the fourth session of the workshop. In this session, panelists discussed long-term impairments and functional limitations that are related to Long COVID, including effects on physical and cognitive functioning, mental health, and quality of life. The final presentation in the session introduced workshop participants to a tool that can be used to assess functioning in COVID-19 patients.

PHYSICAL FUNCTION, COGNITIVE FUNCTION, AND HEALTH-RELATED QUALITY OF LIFE

Laura Tabacof, research instructor at the Department of Rehabilitation and Human Performance at Icahn School of Medicine at Mount Sinai, began by giving a working definition of Long COVID, stating that it refers to a range of new, returning, or ongoing health problems experienced by people 4 or more weeks after initial coronavirus infection. Based on the best available evidence and guidelines, she said, no immunological confirmation (e.g., PCR or antibody test) is required for diagnosis, and there is no well-established biomarker. The umbrella of Long COVID includes other conditions including postintensive care syndrome (PICS), pulmonary fibrosis, myocarditis, postviral syndromes, and worsening of preexisting comorbidities such as asthma. At Mount Sinai, Tabacof and her colleagues developed a patient-reported survey to better understand patients' impairments and rehabilitation needs. This online survey, said Tabacof, was an adaptation of the World Health Organization (WHO) case record form for postacute COVID conditions, and included questions about demographics, past medical history, acute COVID-19 illness, as well as a symptom checklist, and a set of validated tools for collecting patient-reported outcomes, including the following:

- Fatigue Severity Scale (Hernández-Ronquillo et al., 2011; Learmonth et al., 2013; Lerdal and Kottorp, 2011)
- MRC Breathlessness Scale (Stenton, 2008; Williams, 2017)
- EuroQol EQ-5D-5L (EuroQol Research Foundation, n.d.; Herdman et al., 2011)
- Patient Health Questionnaire (PHQ-2) (Arroll et al., 2010; Kroenke et al., 2003)
- General Anxiety Disorder-7 (GAD-7) (Spitzer et al., 2006)
- Neuro-QOL Cognitive Function 8-item Short Form (Neuro-QoL) (Iverson et al., 2021)
- WHO Disability Assessment Schedule [WHODAS] (Üstün et al., 2010).

Using this survey, Tabacof and her colleagues created a preliminary data set of 156 individuals referred to Mount Sinai for postacute COVID-19 care (Tabacof et al., 2022). The majority of patients (107) were female, with an average age of 44. Only about half had a COVID-19 infection confirmed by a PCR or antibody test, and the remainder were considered to have had a probable COVID-19 infection on the basis of the WHO criteria. Only about 10 percent of patients had been hospitalized during the acute phase of their illness. Tabacof described the findings from the study. The most common symptoms reported were fatigue, brain fog, headache, insomnia, dizziness, dyspnea, memory loss, and palpitations. Physical exertion triggered symptom exacerbation for 86 percent of patients, stress did so for 69 percent, and dehydration for 49 percent. "Alarmingly," said Tabacof, COVID-19-related symptoms persisted for a median of 351 days, with a range from 82 to 457 days.

Scores for the study's patient-reported outcomes data revealed that 63 percent had mild cognitive impairment, and 15 percent had severe impairment. In addition, 78 percent had debilitating fatigue and 40 percent had debilitating dyspnea. Self-reported effects on physical function were quantified; Tabacof said there was a large reduction in frequency of both moderate and vigorous physical activity, which is potentially correlated with exacerbation of symptoms after physical exertion. This reduction in activity, she said, raises concerns about the long-term health risks associated with inactivity, and may also be reducing people's ability to work. Over three-quarters of survey respondents were employed full-time before contracting COVID-19; this decreased to 41 percent postacute COVID-19 (Figure 5-1). While some of

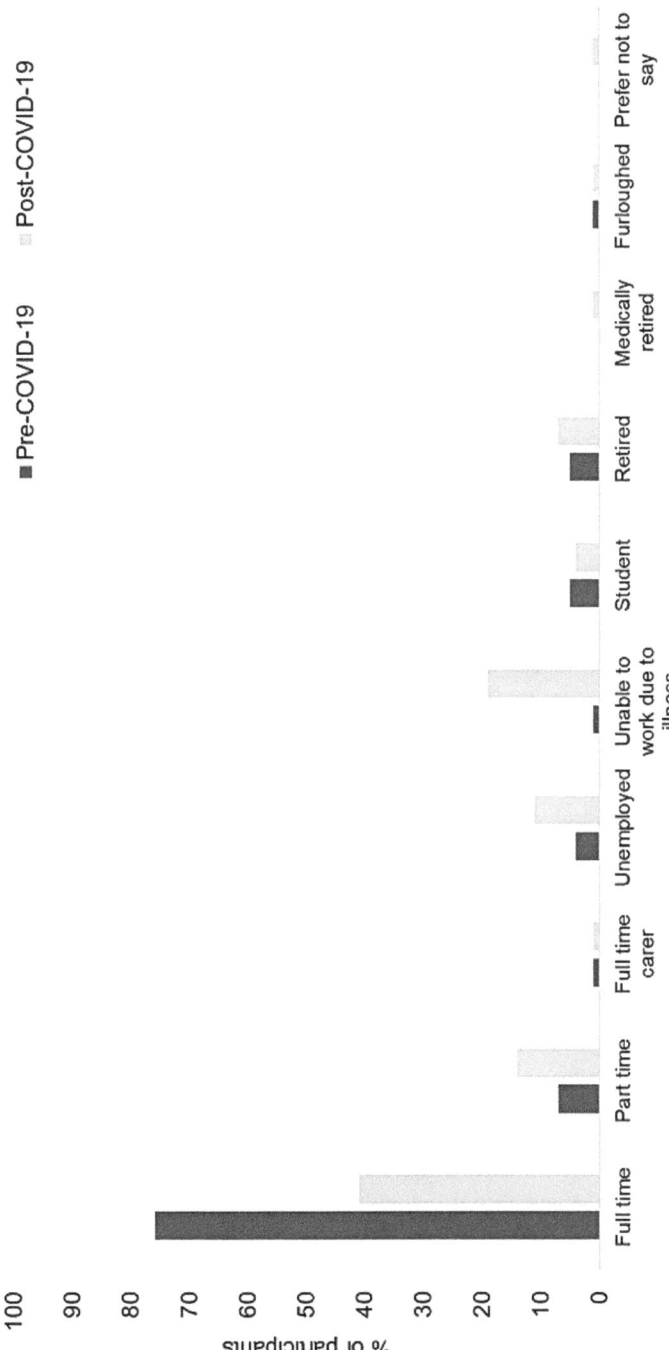

FIGURE 5-1 Full time employment pre- and post-COVID-19.
SOURCE: Tabacof et al., 2022, p. 52, in Laura Tabacof presentation, March 22, 2022.

this decrease may be caused by the economic effects of the pandemic, the high percentage of people who reported being unable to work because of illness suggests significant COVID-19-related disability.

In addition to the survey of 156 individuals, Tabacof also presented unpublished data from a survey she and her colleagues conducted with a larger sample of 533 patients with postacute COVID-19; the majority were female, aged 46 on average, and 90 percent had never been hospitalized for acute COVID-19. Respondents answered the same questions used in the smaller sample, addressing fatigue, cognitive impairment, and disability. Using the Fatigue Severity Scale (FSS), 81 percent had scores indicating severe fatigue, with a mean score of 5.4 out of 7. Placed in context with other conditions, said Tabacof, this level of fatigue is comparable to other postviral syndromes, and more severe than levels of fatigue in other chronic neurological conditions (e.g., multiple sclerosis) or in the general population.

On the Neuro QOL Cognitive Function scale, 70 percent of respondents indicated some level of dysfunction, with 51 percent reporting moderate to severe dysfunction (Figure 5-2). In contrast, about 20 percent of the general population is estimated to have moderate to severe cognitive dysfunction (HealthMeasures, n.d.; Iverson et al., 2021), she said. Tabacof emphasized that the postacute COVID-19 cohort was generally younger than the general population, so the difference in cognitive dysfunction may be even greater.

The EuroQol-5D-5L is a self-reported instrument that measures health-related quality of life on a five-component scale: mobility, usual activities, depression/anxiety, self-care, and pain/discomfort. Using this instrument, Tabacof and her colleagues found that over half of the post-acute COVID-19 cohort had moderate, severe, or extreme problems in the areas of usual activities, and just under 50 percent had moderate, severe, or extreme pain/discomfort (Figure 5-3). Anxiety and depression were also measured using the GAD-7 and PHQ-2. Tabacof observed that the exact effect of COVID-19 on mental health is complex to estimate, but these data suggest the levels of anxiety and depression in patients with Long COVID are not that different from normative or baseline values. This, she added, is in contrast to the data on fatigue and cognitive dysfunction, which were notably different from the norm.

Respondents were asked questions about the effect of COVID-19 on their employment status. One-third indicated they were unable to work the same number of hours because of their health, while a quarter were unable to work at all because of their health (Figure 5-4). Of the 217 people who answered a question about disability insurance, 17 had applied, and 7 were approved. Scores on the WHODAS instrument to assess disability demonstrated that more than half of respondents reported some level of disability and about a quarter reported severe or extreme disability, said Tabacof.

LONG-TERM IMPAIRMENTS AND FUNCTIONAL LIMITATIONS 57

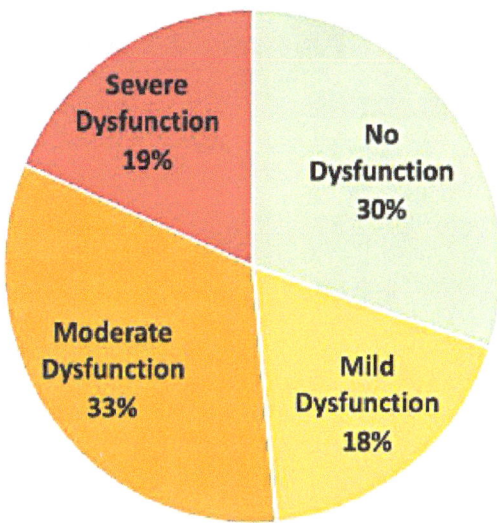

FIGURE 5-2 Neuro QOL Cognitive Function scale scores among patients with post-acute COVID-19 infection.
SOURCE: Laura Tabacof presentation, March 22, 2022; unpublished data from the speaker.

In concluding, Tabacof identified five main points from this research:

- Long COVID can reduce function and participation for longer than 12 months, regardless of the severity of acute illness.
- Impairments are comparable or more severe than what is seen in other work-debilitating conditions.
- With no universal biomarker for Long COVID or related disability, diagnosis should be based on patient-reported symptoms or outcomes and clinical evaluation.
- Clinicians should be trained to diagnose Long COVID so prevalence can be determined and proper care can be delivered.
- Investment in local support systems of Long COVID is crucial: rehabilitation, care delivery workforce, and infrastructure.

LIMITATIONS AND IMPAIRMENTS AFTER A STAY IN THE INTENSIVE CARE UNIT

Postintensive care syndrome (PICS) is a well-established condition that affects survivors and families after a stay in the intensive care unit (ICU), said Alba Azola, rehabilitation physician and codirector of the Post-Acute COVID-

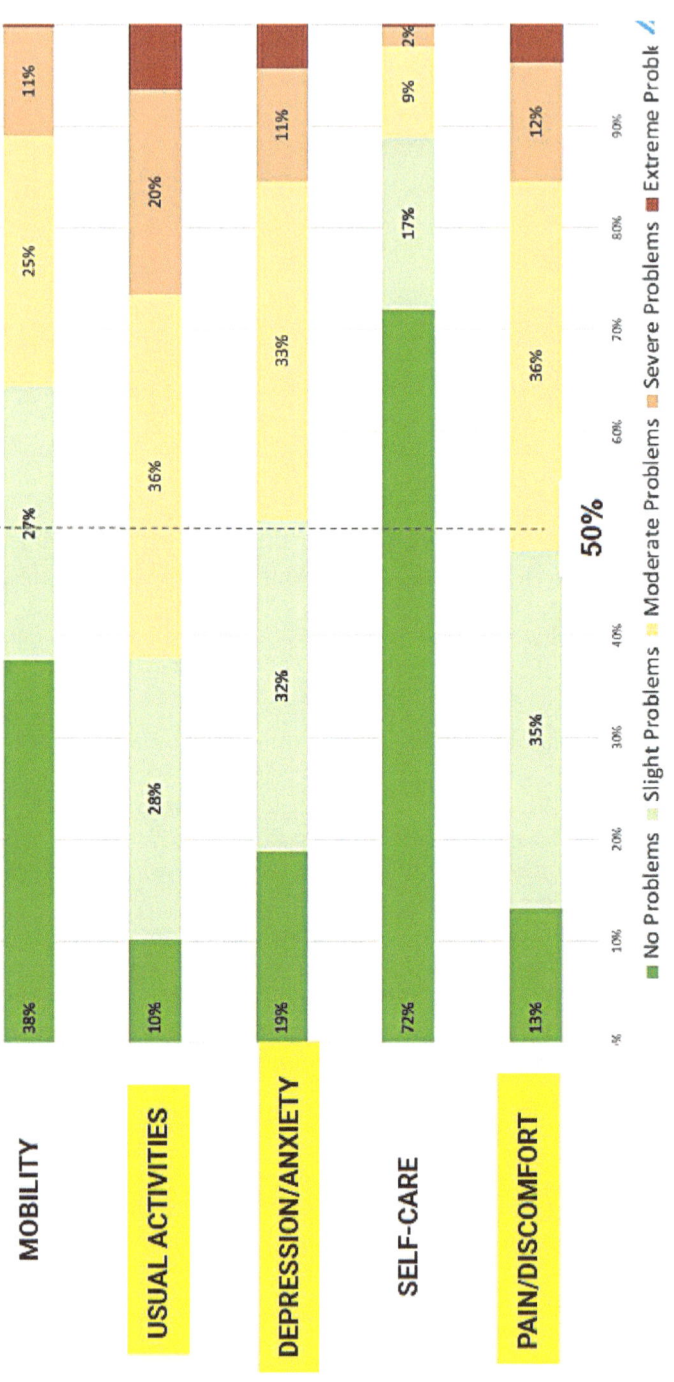

FIGURE 5-3 Health-related quality of life on the EuroQol-5D-5L scale among patients with postacute COVID-19 infection.
SOURCE: Laura Tabacof presentation, March 22, 2022; unpublished data from the speaker.

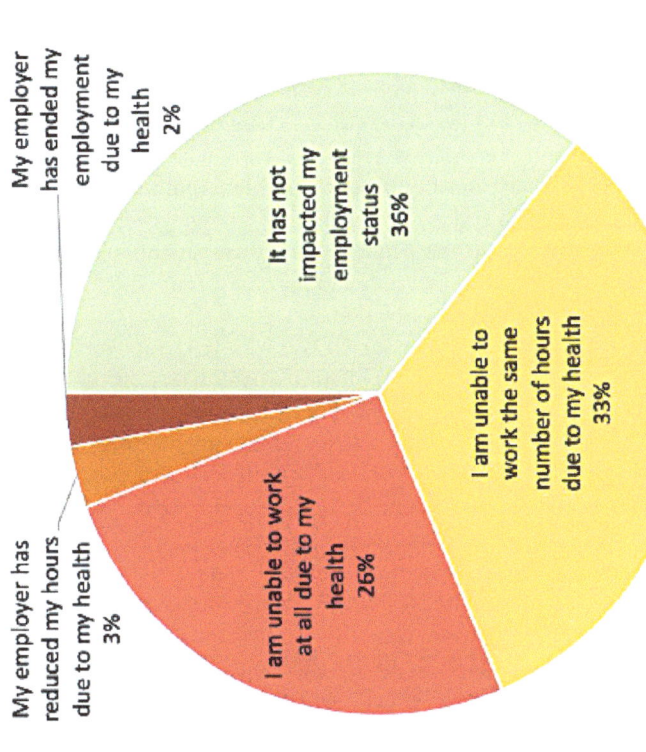

FIGURE 5-4 Employment status among patients with postacute COVID-19 infection.
SOURCE: Laura Tabacof presentation, March 22, 2022; unpublished data from the speaker.

19 Team at Johns Hopkins Hospital. The knowledge about this condition can be used to inform the expected outcomes for patients who were in the ICU with acute, severe COVID-19, she said. PICS affects patients in three main areas: mental health, including anxiety, PTSD, and depression; cognitive impairments, including executive function, memory, attention, visuospatial ability, and mental processing speed; and physical impairments, including pulmonary, neuromuscular, and physical function. The family of the survivor may deal with issues of anxiety, PTSD, depression, and complicated grief.

A 2003 study (Herridge et al., 2003) looked at outcomes over time for ICU patients with acute respiratory distress syndrome (ARDS), said Azola. The study found that patients lost about 20 percent of body weight by the time they were discharged, and although they regained most of the weight, the lean muscle tissue that was lost was replaced with fat. Using the 6-minute walk test to measure mobility, patients improved over time but were still below baseline by 12 months. Only half had returned to work at 12 months, and of these, a quarter could not return to their original job or required modifications. Physical impairments included muscle wasting and weakness, foot drop, and joint immobility.

Patients admitted to the ICU during the COVID-19 pandemic experienced a number of environmental and management differences that may worsen their outcomes, said Alba in discussing an analysis of studies (Parker et al., 2021) (Figure 5-5). These patients spent a longer time on mechanical ventilation and experienced frequent position changes; these experiences can worsen myopathy and put patients at risk for peripheral nerve injuries and brachial plexopathies. Mental health and cognition could be worsened by prolonged ICU stays with visitor restrictions, media coverage of the pandemic, and anxiety and grief about the pandemic. Further, patients may have had reduced access to rehabilitation services and may have dealt with fear of infection, lifestyle changes, and social isolation.

Evidence about the outcomes for COVID-19 ICU survivors is beginning to emerge, said Azola. Observed physical impairments include shoulder subluxation, brachial plexus injuries, peripheral nerve injuries, and joint contractures. One study (Wiertz et al., 2021) found that upon admission to acute in-patient rehabilitation, nearly 73 percent of patients had muscle weakness, 13 percent had foot drop, and about 22 percent demonstrated limited range of motion in joints. There was a high risk of dysphagia, with 40 percent of patients admitted to the rehabilitation center still requiring feeding tubes or adapted consistency for meals. Nearly 75 percent of patients still required supplemental oxygen. In terms of cognitive impairment, said Azola, COVID-19 patients who were in the ICU have significantly more impairment than COVID-19 patients who were either not hospitalized or hospitalized but not in the ICU. Mental health was also impaired, with significant propor-

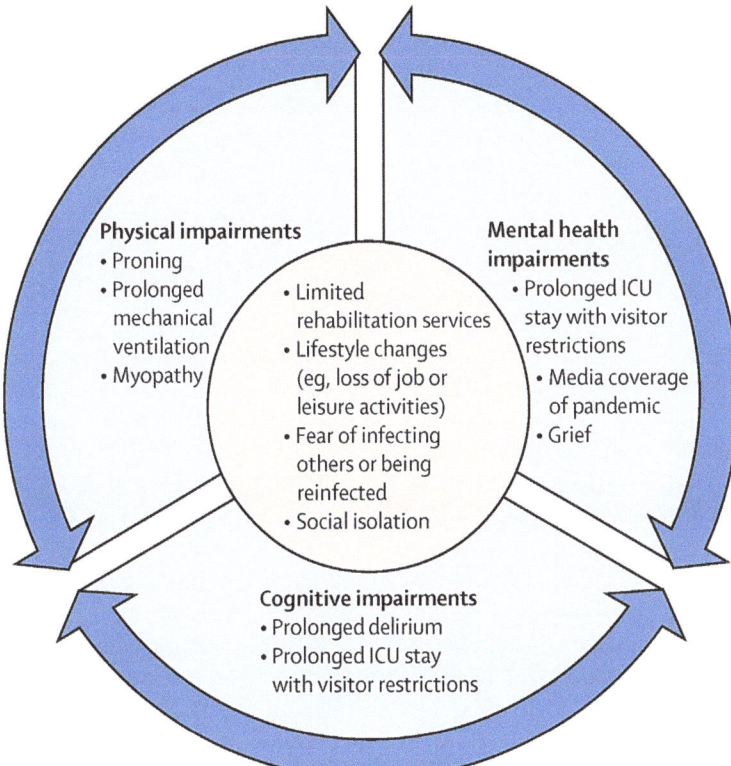

FIGURE 5-5 COVID-19 pandemic-related factors that could exacerbate physical, cognitive, or mental health impairments.
SOURCE: Reprinted from Lancet Respiratory Medicine 9(11), Parker et al., 2021, p. 1331, with permission from Elsevier, in Alba Azola presentation, March 22, 2022.

tions of patients reporting psychiatric distress, functional decline, anxiety, and depression.

Azola summarized her main points:

- A hospital stay in the intensive care unit is associated with physical, cognitive, and mental health impairments that may lead to long-term disability. In one study, more than half the patients were unable to return to work at 12-months.
- Pandemic-related factors can place COVID-19 patients who were in the ICU at greater risk for physical, cognitive, or mental health impairments; limitations on activity; or restrictions on social participation, and thus be at higher risk of long-term disability.

MENTAL HEALTH EFFECTS

As other speakers have discussed, Long COVID patients may have an increased risk of poor mental health outcomes, said Monica Kurylo, professor and director of the Division of Psychology at the University of Kansas Medical Center. These outcomes include diagnoses such as anxiety, depression, PTSD, obsessive-compulsive disorder (OCD), and panic attacks, as well as such symptoms as sleep problems, substance abuse, distress, and low quality of life. The time course of mental health issues in COVID-19 patients is unclear, said Kurylo, and more research is needed in this area. Most studies of mental health have measured outcomes about 4 or 6 months after a COVID-19 diagnosis, while fewer studies measure outcomes at 12 months after acute COVID-19 illness. It is also unclear at this point whether and to what extent mental health symptoms are related to the severity and duration of the acute COVID-19 illness.

As others have mentioned, said Kurylo, it is challenging to untangle the mental health effects of COVID-19 illness from the effects of the pandemic in general. COVID-19 can exacerbate preexisting mental health conditions and can also contribute to new diagnoses and symptoms. For example, sleep problems and substance abuse may exacerbate each other as well as affect other mental and physical symptoms. Other COVID-19-related factors may also affect and be affected by mental health, including grief, loss of family members, financial concerns, racial and ethnic disparities, and community stressors.

Screening for and evaluation of mental health symptoms can be conducted using a variety of tools, said Kurylo, including the Patient Health Questionnaire (PHQ-2) (Kroenke et al., 2003), the Geriatric Depression Scale (Sheikh and Yesavage, 1986), the Beck Depression Inventory (Beck et al., 1988), and the Epworth Sleepiness Scale (Johns, 1991). Treatments depend on the needs and interests of the patients, noted Kurylo, and can include individual therapy, cognitive behavioral therapy, mindfulness training, group therapy, Long COVID support groups, peer support, phone and computer apps, and alternative approaches such as biofeedback and meditation.

CHILD AND ADOLESCENT FUNCTIONING

Children and adolescents have experienced COVID-19 differently than adults in a number of ways, said Alicia Johnston, instructor at Harvard Medical School and codirector of the Multidisciplinary Post-COVID-19 Program at Boston Children's Hospital. Children are far less likely to have severe disease and to be hospitalized than adults. Most children who develop Long COVID, she said, had mild or even asymptomatic infections. Children generally have fewer comorbidities and are usually previously healthy; because of this, the symptoms of Long COVID can be a significant departure from baseline for children and families. Young children or those with developmental delays may not be able to articulate their symptoms or concerns, which makes diagnosis of Long COVID more challenging; pediatricians have to rely on histories from people such as parents and teachers to guide treatment and management.

The prevalence of Long COVID in children is unknown, said Johnston, with estimates ranging widely. Earlier in the pandemic, studies suggested that somewhere between 8 and 52 percent of children with confirmed SARS-CoV-2 infections would develop Long COVID (Borch et al., 2022; Buonsenso et al., 2021; Ludvigsson et al., 2021; Say et al., 2021; Zimmermann et al., 2021).

Later studies that included healthy control groups had lower estimates of between 0.8 and 2 percent (Borch et al., 2022; Molteni et al., 2021; Radtke et al., 2021). Children under 5 seem to be less frequently affected and have fewer symptoms than older children and adolescents (Borch et al., 2022; Molteni et al., 2021; Say et al., 2021), although Johnston noted that these children may be less able to communicate their symptoms well. Like in adults, a variety of symptoms have been reported in children that have been attributed to Long COVID, including fatigue, postexertional fatigue, exercise intolerance, dyspnea, cough, dizziness, brain fog, insomnia, muscle weakness, pain, nausea, and anosmia. It is important to note, however, that many of these symptoms are nonspecific and highly prevalent in the general population. In fact, said Johnston, studies that included healthy controls found many children in the control group complaining of ongoing symptoms similar to those reported in the Long COVID group. This begs the question of which symptoms are actually caused by SARS-CoV-2 infection and which might be caused by other factors such as the stress and social isolation of the pandemic.

Johnston gave an overview of the studies on Long COVID that have been conducted in the pediatric population. Far less data are available on children, she said, in part because early in the pandemic there was a focus on higher-risk populations. A 2021 review article (Zimmermann et al., 2021) examined 14 studies of Long COVID in children, and found major limitations in nearly all the studies, including lack of clear case definitions, absence of control groups, low follow-up rates, small sample sizes, reliance on symptom reports without clinical assessment, and multiple types of selection and information biases. Our understanding of Long COVID in children "really lags behind our adult counterparts and underscores the need for well-designed studies with appropriate controls," she said.

There are many varied potential effects and long-term challenges for children with Long COVID, said Johnston. These include effects on mental health, school absenteeism and performance, social activities, and parental stress and employment, all of which could have long-term consequences. For example, school nonattendance has been associated with adverse health and social outcomes in both the short and long term, said Johnston. The effects of Long COVID may be particularly acute for children from socioeconomically disadvantaged backgrounds and ethnic minority groups, further exacerbating existing disparities.

The lack of data and the fact that the pandemic began relatively recently makes it difficult to predict the likely outcomes for children with symptoms of Long COVID. While most studies do not have a long follow-up period, they generally show a decrease in the number of symptomatic patients and the burden of the disease over time. Our understanding of other conditions may also be useful in understanding the trajectory of Long COVID, said Johnston. For example, a study on ME/CFS in adolescents found that half reported severe fatigue and physical impairment at 2 years postdiagnosis, and that school and work attendance in the population was low (van Geelan et al., 2010). An older study of 35 adolescents found that 20 percent had ongoing significant symptoms and activity limitation at 13 years after the onset of symptoms (Bell, 2001).

As of March 2022, almost 12.8 million children in the United States have tested positive for COVID-19 (American Academy of Pediatrics, 2022), said Johnston. Using the lower prevalence estimates of 0.8 percent to 2 percent of children developing Long COVID, somewhere between 100,000 and 250,000 children will be affected, she said. If the persistence of Long COVID is similar to ME/CFS, between 20,000 and 50,000 children will enter adulthood with ongoing health needs. However, she said that these numbers are likely an underestimation of the burden of disease. The CDC has reported that around 75 percent of children in the United States have likely been infected with SARS-CoV-2 (Clarke et al., 2022),[1] and these numbers continue to grow.

Johnston shared final thoughts:

- Children may experience significant long-term physical, cognitive, social, and emotional limitations because of Long COVID.
- Early recognition and treatment of symptoms and support of return to school and other activities with appropriate accommodations is essential to the overall recovery of children.
- Identification of family stressors (e.g., financial, housing, employment, safety, social isolation) and availability of support systems may provide emotional and logistical support and guide medical therapies.
- Areas of further research include understanding the long-term effect of Long COVID on children as they transition into adulthood is needed.

---

[1] The speaker updated this information after the workshop.

CLINFIT COVID-19: A NOVEL TOOL TO ASSESS FUNCTIONING

Gerold Stucki, professor and chair of the Department of Health Sciences and Medicine at the University of Lucerne, introduced workshop participants to ClinFIT COVID-19. ClinFIT (Clinical Functioning Information Tool) is a clinical measure that can be tailored to specific population needs and is based on the WHO's International Classification of Functioning, Disability, and Health (ICF), said Stucki. ClinFIT COVID-19 is being developed in collaboration with the International Society of Physical and Rehabilitation Medicine (Frontera et al., 2019). The ICF is a framework that captures a wide range of a health condition's implications, including body functions and structures, limitations on activities, environmental factors, and personal factors (Figure 5-6). Using this framework, ClinFIT COVID-19 is being developed as a way to assess people's lived experience in the clinical context, he said.

There are a number of advantages of using an ICF-based approach, said Stucki. It is an established and internationally recognized reference system for clinical measurement and the standardized reporting of functioning information. The list of functioning domains is mutually exclusive and cumulatively exhaustive. Clinical measures can be tailored in rapid response to public health emergencies, such as COVID-19. Functioning information can be reported independent of the data collection tool or the data source, and data can be easily compared.

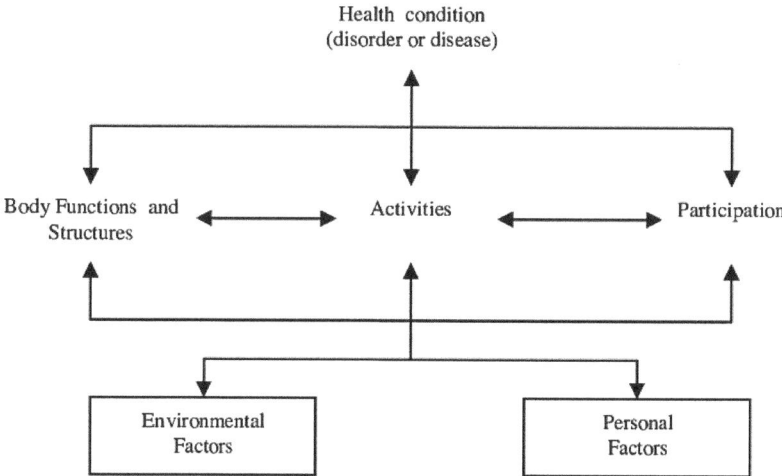

FIGURE 5-6 International Classification of Functioning, Disability, and Health model of functioning and disability.
SOURCE: Reproduced from *International Classification of Functioning, Disability and Health*, WHO, 2001, p. 18, in Gerold Stucki presentation, March 22, 2022.

The first step in the development of this tool, said Stucki, was to identify the functioning domains that matter to people living with Long COVID; this was done through a network of international collaboration. The next step, which is ongoing, is to validate the set of domains in a broader population. Stucki presented the domains that have been identified (Table 5-1). The domains include things that matter to patients, such as pain, emotion, energy, and sleep. Other functional measures include carrying out daily routines, walking, and employment. Stucki said these are universally agreed on measures that can be referred to by anyone in the world.

The next step, he said, is a system for using the tool in clinical practice and collecting the data. The functioning domains are simple descriptions of ICF categories, and experts rate functioning limitations based on all available information (e.g., patient history, patient-reported outcomes, and clinical examinations). Raters can use a 1–10 numeric scale, a 0–4 numeric scale, or a 0–4 scale with specifications. These different scales can then be transferred to a 0–100 scale for statistical purposes. The confidence intervals for each domain depend on the area being measured.

In closing, Stucki reiterated three main points:

- An ICF-based approach can support clinical measurement and standardized reporting of functioning information.
- COVID-19 affects a broad spectrum of functioning domains ranging from body functions to activities and participation.
- ClinFIT COVID-19 is a customizable and easy-to-use clinical measure that captures what matters to people with COVID-19.

DISCUSSION

Malone moderated a question-and-answer session with panelists and workshop participants.

Is there a set of tests or outcome measures that would be useful to SSA in making disability determinations for patients with Long COVID? Is it possible or necessary to look for a biomarker or other definitive signal of Long COVID?

The first step in measuring the effect of Long COVID, said Stucki, is to carefully define *what* needs to be measured; that is, identify the important domains, including body function and activity limitations. Depending on the domain, different types of tools can be used for measurement, including patient-reported outcome measures, clinical tests, or rating systems. Kurylo added that it is important to use consistent measures to evaluate effect; she noted that measures that are publicly available online can be useful for patients to monitor themselves. There is a complexity to the presentation of Long

TABLE 5-1 ClinFIT COVID-19 Categories

ICF category (code and title) and corresponding simple description	Acute (n=13)	Postacute (n=15)	Longterm (n=16)
b130 Energy and drive functions (G): Psychological energy and motivational drive to move towards goals, satisfy needs and control impulses	√	√	√
b134 Sleep functions: Cycle, quality, and amount of sleep	√	√	√
b140 Attention functions: ICF book: Specific mental functions focusing on external stimulus or internal experience for the required period of time	√	√	
b152 Emotional functions (G): Mental functions for the modulation of the expression of feelings and emotions	√	√	√
b280 Sensation of pain (G): Unpleasant sensation indicating potential or actual damage of some body structure	√	√	√
b440 Respiratory functions: ICF book: Functions of inhaling air into the lungs, the exchange of gases between air and blood, and exhaling	√	√	√
b445 Respiratory muscle functions: ICF book: Functions of the muscles involved in breathing air	√	√	√
b455 Exercise tolerance functions: Capacity of enduring physical exertion related to respiratory and cardiovascular functions	√	√	√
b710 Mobility of joint functions: Range and ease of movement of a joint	√	√	√
b730 Muscle power functions: Capacity to generate force through the contraction of a muscle or muscle groups	√	√	√

continued

TABLE 5-1 Continued

ICF category (code and title) and corresponding simple description	Acute (n=13)	Postacute (n=15)	Longterm (n=16)
d230 Carrying out daily routine (G): Plan, manage and complete routine daily life activities	√	√	√
d240 Handling stress and other psychological demands: Manage and control the psychological demands to carry out tasks demanding responsibilities involving stress and/or distractions and/or critical issues	√	√	√
d450 Walking (G): Moving in an upright position, step by step, always maintaining a support on the ground	√	√	√
d455 Moving around (G): Moving around differently from walking (for example running, going up and down the stairs, jumping, climbing, swimming, etc.)		√	√
d850 Remunerative employment (G): Properly performing remunerative employment (full or part time or self-employed) in all its aspects			√
d920 Recreation and leisure: Engaging in recreational or leisure activity (play, cultural and sports activities etc., during spare time)			√
s430 Structure of the respiratory system: ICF book: Trachea, lungs, thoracic cage, muscles of respiration		√	√

NOTE: Large check symbol = initially proposed categories; Small check symbol = additional categories selected using a multistep process; G = Generic-7 category; ICF = International Classification of Functioning, Disability, and Health.
SOURCE: Selb et al., 2021, p. 182, in Gerold Stucki presentation, March 22, 2022.

COVID, said Azola, and it would be difficult to find one "magic" test. It is a complex syndrome that has multiple facets and affects individuals in different ways; for this reason, it is more useful to look at integrated functional domains to view the patient within the context of their individual impairments and environment. Johnston added that different biomarkers for Long COVID, such as microbiome status, cytokine levels, immunoglobulin levels, are the subject of current research. But, regardless of whether a biomarker exists, she said that what is important from a clinical standpoint is comprehensively evaluating a patient's dysfunction and determining how to support them.

SSA has a responsibility to accurately and efficiently evaluate claimants while being good stewards of public funds. Is there research to support the validity of patient-reported measures as compared to clinical measures? What are the limitations of patient-reported measures, and are there ways to overcome them?

"It is always going to be a challenge to know for sure the extent to which any given person is giving an accurate assessment of their symptoms," said Kurylo. We have to place our trust in the patient, and can also rely on the input of loved ones who are observing the patient and seeing how a condition is affecting him or her. Azola shared a perspective from her clinic, saying that they perform objective tests of cognitive dysfunction, and also conduct subjective testing to measure the patient's perceived level of dysfunction. She said depressed patients tend to perceive more impairment in cognition than the objective test reveals, but that there is "definitely a component of cognitive dysfunction that is separate from their depression and anxiety and post-traumatic stress."

Tabacof noted that while there are limitations of patient-reported outcomes, including subjectivity and risk of recall bias, there are also limitations of biomarker or clinical testing. There is no universal test or set of tests to diagnose or quantify the effect of Long COVID, and it is unknown if existing tests correlate objectively with levels of impairment. Further, if clinical testing is required for diagnosis of Long COVID, there is a potential to exacerbate health care disparities because of lack of access to testing. Johnston added that certain objective tests—such as neuropsychiatric testing—can be difficult to get conducted in a timely manner, particularly during the pandemic. The current best practice, said Tabacof, is to rely on informed clinical evaluation to identify a cluster of symptoms that is compatible with a diagnosis of Long COVID, and to not use objective laboratory or imaging findings as the only measure of a patient's well-being.

Is there any way to predict what percentage of people, or which specific individuals, might be unable to work 12 months after an acute COVID-19 infection?

Tabacof replied that this is an important area but not one that she has objective data on at this point. She and her colleagues are analyzing their data about employment to examine whether employment outcomes correlate with other functional assessments and disability level. Kurylo added that while this question is challenging to answer right now, she hopes that this workshop will spur additional research in this area.

What has been learned about the relationship between neurological issues and mental health in Long COVID?

It can be difficult to separate neurological and psychiatric conditions because neurological issues can produce psychiatric symptoms, said Kurylo. While it is important to recognize that there can be a relationship between the two, the critical thing is to address the symptoms in a well-rounded and effective way. Pre-COVID-19 research indicates that the best and longest-lasting mental health treatments are typically a combination of psychotherapy and medication, said Kurylo, and there is reason to hope that this would be the same for Long COVID patients who are experiencing mental health symptoms.

One of the essential requirements of work is the ability to follow instructions with reasonable consistency; is there evidence that Long COVID particularly compromises this ability?

Tabacof said that she and her colleagues are currently conducting data analyses to determine how functional outcomes such as cognitive function, anxiety, and depression affect employment. Azola added that her research has found that some Long COVID patients may have difficulty acquiring new skills or new information. In addition, recall and verbal fluency may be affected, as well as spatial reasoning. For example, some patients have difficulty navigating computer systems that they were familiar with and worked with for several years prior to contracting COVID-19.

SSA typically uses psychological testing (e.g. Wechsler memory scales) to determine the severity or degree of limitations brought on by a mental health impairment. Will these tools continue to remain valid and effective in assessing impairments related to Long COVID?

Kurylo responded that these types of tests are likely to remain useful in assessing Long COVID patients. In her experience, she said, these tests can be helpful for determine the strengths of Long COVID patients, as well as the challenges. Even with the tests, however, assessment still requires gathering information about changes over time and a degree of speculation about which symptoms are related to Long COVID. Azola said that some of the tests for cognitive performance can be very lengthy, some taking 2 or 3 hours. She has noticed that the length of the test can affect some patients' performances. Tabacof agreed, and added that some patients are unable to complete a lengthy test, and that doing so can exacerbate their symptoms. Further, said Azola, test performance can fluctuate from day to day, depending on the patient's symptoms and how well they are being managed. Azola noted that this fluctuation can occur with both psychological and cognitive testing, as well as physical tests such as those for orthostatic intolerance.

6

Clinical Practices and System Approaches for Improving Health and Recovery from Long COVID

Monica Verduzco-Gutierrez, professor and chair of the Department of Rehabilitation Medicine at the University of Texas Health San Antonio, introduced the final panel of the workshop, which examined clinical practices and system approaches for improving health and recovery from Long COVID. In this session, speakers described and explored systematic issues pertaining to Long COVID, and discussed how guidance statements, care models, and policy can help to improve care for patients with Long COVID.

CLINICAL GUIDANCE STATEMENTS

Steven Flanagan, professor and chair of rehabilitation medicine and medical director of Rusk Rehabilitation at NYU Langone Health, shared the experiences of the American Academy of Physical Medicine and Rehabilitation (AAPM&R) in developing and disseminating guidance on Long COVID for its members. AAPM&R represents about 10,000 physiatrists, who are medical doctors specializing in disability and function. Physiatrists treat disability and impairments that result from injury or disease in nearly every organ system, he said, which makes them uniquely qualified to deal with Long COVID. About a year ago, AAPM&R called on President Biden's administration and Congress to put together a plan of action to deal with the public health crisis of Long COVID, said Flanagan. With upwards of 24 million people experiencing or having experienced symptoms of Long COVID (American Academy of Physical Medicine and Rehabilitation, 2022), the resources, infrastructure, and providers to deliver necessary care are needed, with focus on ensuring equity in care and equal access to care, regardless of race, ethnicity, socioeconomic status, gender, sexual orientation, or other characteristics, said Flanagan. The call to action had an effect, said Flanagan, with the National Institutes of Health and the Biden Administration making strides toward delivering the resources necessary.

Flanagan told workshop participants about AAPM&R's efforts in this area. Together with Johns Hopkins, AAPM&R developed a dashboard that shows estimated PASC cases by state and county. The dashboard uses an assumption that 10 to 30 percent of adults who survived COVID-19 will continue to have symptoms at 6 months postinfection (American Academy of Physical Medicine and Rehabilitation, 2022). In March 2021, AAPM&R assembled a collaborative of providers, patients, caregivers, and representatives from post-COVID clinics. The PASC Collaborative's goals are to delineate existing best practices, disseminate lessons learned, and develop resources for primary care providers and PASC clinics.

The PASC Collaborative is multidisciplinary, and its leadership includes specialists in physiatry, population health, pulmonary medicine, and critical care. Patients and caregivers are important to the collaborative because they are "in the trenches," said Flanagan; their experiences provide valuable insight for guidance statements. Collaborative members also include representatives from 35 post-COVID clinics, such as physicians, rehabilitation professionals, psychologists, and others. The collaborative uses a systematic process for the development of guidance statements and involves an equity subcommittee to ensure that the statements address equal access and care for subpopulations.

Thus far, the PASC Collaborative has published guidance statements on cognitive symptoms, breathing discomfort and respiratory sequelae, and fatigue.[1] The statements, said Flanagan, are based on the experience and expertise of people working and living in the world of Long COVID. Some of the evidence available is from conditions similar to PASC, but the guidance statements primarily integrate current experience with the limited evidence available for assessing and managing Long COVID. Guidance statements are published on a rolling basis. Guidance statements in development will address cardiac impairment, pediatric Long COVID, and autonomic dysfunction; future topics include headache and vertigo. Flanagan emphasized that developing guidance is an iterative process because evidence about the etiology, assessment, and risks for Long COVID is just beginning to emerge. While this process will continue for years, he said, it is critical to get guidance out to the providers and clinics who are treating patients right now.

---

[1] PASC Collaborative Guidance statements: https://www.aapmr.org/members-publications/covid-19/multidisciplinary-quality-improvement-initiative (accessed May 19, 2022).

INTEGRATED CARE MODEL: ADULT POPULATION

Integrated care, said Benjamin Abramoff, assistant professor of physical medicine and rehabilitation and director of the Post-COVID Assessment and Recovery Clinic at the University of Pennsylvania, is a system of care that focuses across the whole spectrum of illness and addresses the health needs of the whole person. Usually a team-based approach that includes providers from multiple specialties, as well as care providers and families, integrated care models have been used in multiple complex conditions, including spinal cord injury, hemophilia, multiple sclerosis, and stroke. This is a beneficial model for Long COVID for a number of reasons, said Abramoff. Individuals who have survived COVID-19 may have significant deficits in physical and cognitive functioning and worsened quality of life. They often have a feeling that they are being "shuffled from provider to provider," and lack a home in the medical system. Because patients may experience symptoms in many different domains, they are sometimes unsure of where to go or who to talk to. Abramoff shared that he has heard from many patients that their provider ordered a few tests and then told them "there is nothing wrong with you." Clinical expertise in Long COVID is lacking; providers are gaining experience, but the knowledge gap is still an ongoing challenge.

Several organizations, said Abramoff, recommend integrated care for Long COVID including the National Institute for Health and Care Excellence (NICE) and CDC. For example, interim guidance from CDC states:

> Health care professionals may also consider referral to multidisciplinary post-COVID-19 care centers, where available, for additional care considerations. Multidisciplinary post-COVID care centers based in a single physical location can provide a comprehensive and coordinated treatment approach to COVID-19 aftercare. (CDC, 2021a)

Abramoff and his colleagues conducted a survey of post-COVID clinics to see how integrated care models have been implemented at different locations (Dundumalla et al., 2022). The survey was completed in May 2021; 45 clinics in 25 states participated. Most of the clinics were homed in physical medicine and rehabilitation, but a high percentage of clinics were also homed in pulmonology and internal medicine. All clinics were multidisciplinary to some extent, said Abramoff, but there was wide variation in the number of specialties routinely involved, the number that are part of the team, and the number that are available during the initial patient visit (Figure 6-1). Around half hold regular, formal interdisciplinary team meetings; Abramoff noted that specialists may be communicating through other channels as well. Abramoff shared a few other interesting findings from the survey. Just over half of clinics directly managed the behavioral health needs of their patients, a third hosted

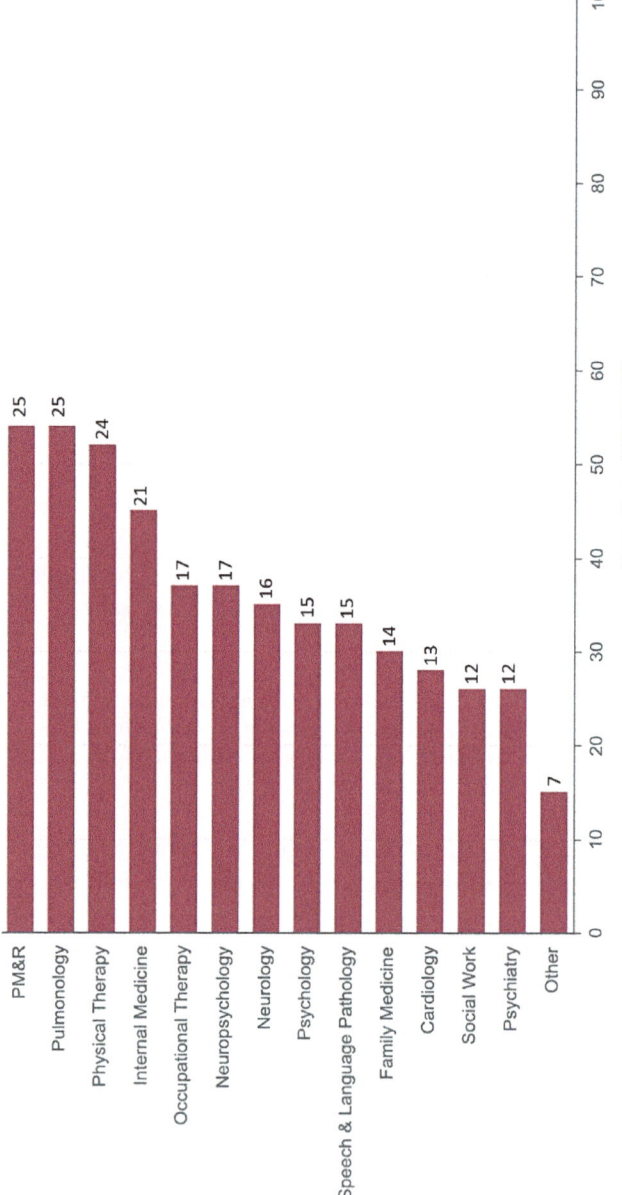

FIGURE 6-1 Specialties available during the initial patient visit in post-COVID clinics.
NOTE: PM&R = physical medicine and rehabilitation.
SOURCE: Benjamin Abramoff presentation, March 22, 2022, based on data from Dundumalla et al., 2022, p. 352, © 2022 American Academy of Physical Medicine and Rehabilitation.

support groups, about two-thirds completed disability paperwork, and almost a quarter reported that they needed more help with staffing, physicians, or case management support. All clinics have processes to involve multiple specialties, and most routinely involve specialties rather than using a hub-and-spoke model. Physical therapy, pulmonology, physical medicine and rehabilitation, neurology, and cardiology are involved in the treatment team in over two-thirds of the clinics.

Abramoff shared his experiences at the Penn Medicine Post-COVID Assessment and Recovery Clinic. The clinic is centered in physical medicine and rehabilitation, and the team has a background in taking care of patients with multisystem, complex medical issues. The team includes a case manager who often is part of the initial patient visit, and they use the hub-and-spoke model to connect with other specialists and providers. The clinic has developed an algorithm that is based on the most common complaints and charts a path to address them using an interdisciplinary method (Figure 6-2).

Abramoff summarized his main points:

- Integrated care is a potential method to improve the care of individuals with Long COVID.
- Numerous integrated care models have been implemented.
- These models can be resource intensive and require significant coordination between providers.
- No research yet suggests if one model is more effective than others.

INTEGRATED CARE MODEL: PEDIATRIC POPULATION

As of March 10, 2022, said Amanda Morrow, assistant professor of physical medicine and rehabilitation at the Johns Hopkins School of Medicine and codirector of the Pediatric Post-COVID-19 Rehabilitation Clinic at Kennedy Krieger Institute, there have been almost 13 million pediatric cases of COVID-19 in the United States, accounting for almost 20 percent of the total cases (American Academy of Pediatrics, 2022). The good news, she said, is that the rates of hospitalization and death are quite low. However, a subset of children—even those with mild illness—will go on to develop Long COVID. Prevalence estimates of persisting symptoms after COVID-19 infection range widely, between 4 and 66 percent (Zimmerman et al., 2021). Fewer studies have been done in the pediatric population than in the adult population, and most studies have had serious limitations. Even if the prevalence of Long COVID is on the lower end of the estimates, she said, this would still affect a significant number of children in the United States.

Children with Long COVID complain of a variety of symptoms across different organ systems, including symptoms of fatigue, cognitive difficulties,

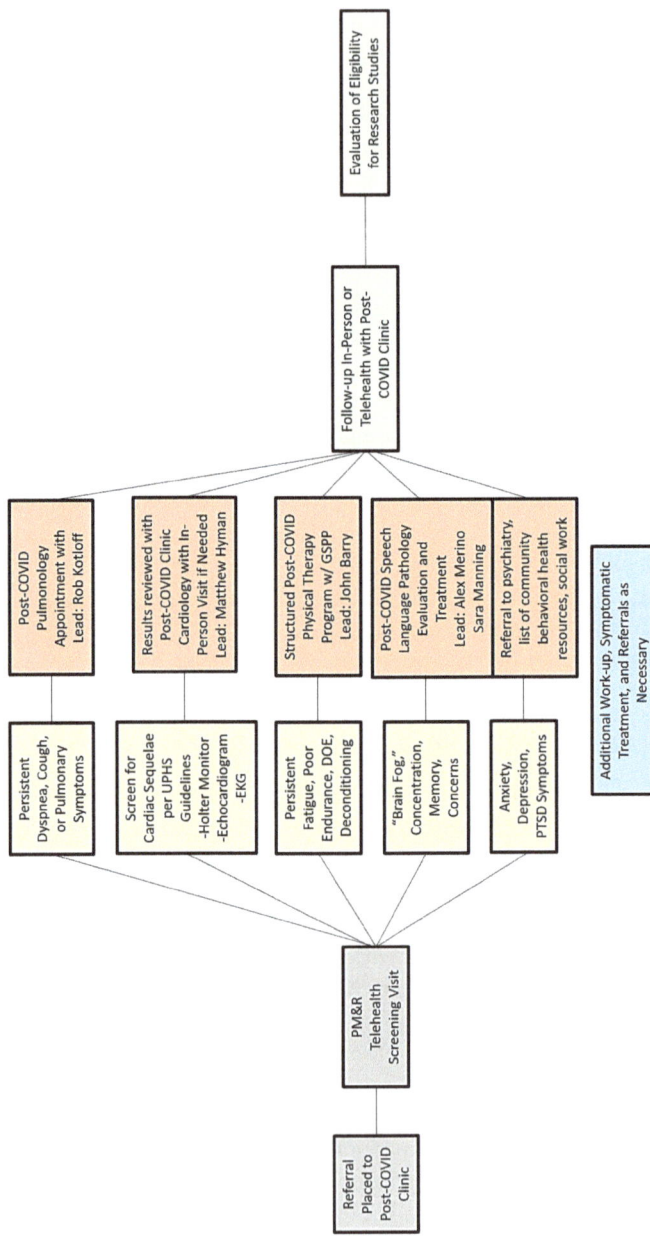

FIGURE 6-2 Algorithm used at Penn Medicine post-COVID clinic for providing care to Long COVID patients.
NOTE: UPHS = University of Pennsylvania Health System; PM&R = physical medicine and rehabilitation; EKG = electrocardiogram; DOE = Department of Education; GSPP = Good Shepherd Penn Partners; PTSD = post-traumatic stress syndrome.
SOURCE: Benjamin Abramoff presentation, March 22, 2022.

mood concerns, headaches, sleep disturbance, dizziness, and lightheadedness. These symptoms are "really impacting the quality of life of our children," and several multidisciplinary clinics have opened to address these symptoms and care for these children. Morrow stated there are currently 11 pediatric Long COVID clinics across the country, as well as 3 clinics specific to MIS-C. There is a history of using the multidisciplinary care model for other complex medical illnesses in both adults and children, including sickle cell disease, traumatic brain injury, pediatric cancers, and cystic fibrosis. The benefits of multidisciplinary specialty clinics include a holistic approach to care, increased communication and coordination, and decreased appointment burden, which can be helpful for disorders with multiple organ system involvement. This approach also has challenges, she said, such as having the institutional infrastructure to support a clinic with adequate space, and managing insurance coverage issues, including limits placed on the number of providers a patient can see in one day. In addition, patient access to clinics and subspecialists vary geographically. Morrow emphasized that multidisciplinary specialty clinics are not designed to take the place of a primary care provider for routine health screening and preventative services, though she said close coordination is essential.

The Kennedy Krieger Institute offers a multidisciplinary, team-based approach that addresses the medical, psychosocial, cognitive, and physical needs of young patients. The goal of the clinic, she said, is to improve patients' overall functioning and ability to participate in their day-to-day tasks, physical activities, school, extracurricular activities, and social engagement. During a patient's initial visit to the clinic, they will be seen by neurology, pediatric physical medicine and rehabilitation, physical therapy, behavioral psychology, and social work. After this visit, the team discusses their assessments and develops a unified treatment plan. Patients can also undergo neuropsychology evaluation, and can meet with an education specialist to develop school-based recommendations. If additional referrals are needed, the clinic has close relationships with specialists who are familiar with Long COVID, and patients can be seen quickly if needed.

For children and adolescents with Long COVID, said Morrow, the emphasis should be on keeping kids in school as much as possible to help normalize their routines, which has educational, psychosocial, and physical benefits. There are accommodations that can help children with Long COVID stay in school and be successful, including planned rest breaks, increased time for testing, and limited assignments. Morrow said it is important to ensure that teachers and staff understand the needs of these children and are able to support them. Adolescents who are transitioning to adulthood could receive care at either an adult or a pediatric clinic, though Morrow suggested that a pediatric clinic may be more appropriate for adolescents who still have school-based concerns.

Morrow and her colleagues have been involved in the development of the AAPM&R guidance statement on pediatric care, which will be coming out shortly. The clinic is also involved in an International Pediatric Post-COVID Condition in Children Collaboration (IP4C) (Brackel et al., 2022), which is currently researching program and clinic models, definitions used, and patient characteristics. The goals of this collaboration, said Morrow, are to develop guidelines, and to create standardized definitions and data harmonization tools to better understand pathophysiology and treatment.

In closing, Morrow highlighted key messages:

- Similar to integrated care models in other complex pediatric illnesses, children with Long COVID may also benefit from multidisciplinary, team-based approaches to care.
- Areas of special consideration include attention to educational needs as well as appropriate transitions of care when reaching adulthood.
- Further research can help determine optimal models of clinical care in pediatric Long COVID.

OVERCOMING BARRIERS TO HEALTH AND SOCIAL INEQUITIES

Zackary Berger, associate professor of medicine at the Johns Hopkins School of Medicine and Johns Hopkins School of Public Health, discussed the disparities and inequities in COVID-19 and Long COVID through the lens of his research with undocumented immigrants in Baltimore. There are a number of vulnerabilities associated with being undocumented (Derose et al., 2007), he said, including limited education, occupational opportunities, and income; limited access to social services; low English proficiency; crowded and poorly maintained residences; stigma and marginalization; involvement with the carceral and/or immigration system; and being overrepresented in the domain of "essential workers." While COVID-19 is a pandemic, said Berger, it can also be seen as a syndemic; that is, the aggregation of the concurrent pandemics of COVID-19, racism and segregation, and socioeconomic inequalities. Each of these pandemics interact and reinforce one another to exacerbate the burden of disease. Berger explained that from a medical anthropology perspective, the COVID-19 pandemic experience embodies the interactions of the individual experience, social aspects of the disease, and the body politic (i.e., the influences of the political and regulatory milieu) (Scheper-Hughes and Lock, 1987).

Berger told workshop participants about his research in Baltimore that focuses on undocumented immigrants' experience with COVID-19. Callers to the Esperanza Center Clinic hotline for COVID-19 information were recruited to participate in a survey; Berger emphasized that this was not a randomized sample but instead a sample enriched in people with COVID-19 experiences in order to understand "how people are actually living through this pandemic." Surveys were conducted in Spanish over the telephone and in interviews from May to July 2021, said Berger. These data are not published at this time, but preliminary results indicate that respondents were often not contacted by the public health department to be notified about exposure, the majority of respondents were concerned about getting care because of their undocumented status, and a plurality of these individuals thought they did not receive adequate medical care when sick with COVID-19.

There are multiple structural factors that worsen symptoms and worsen the effect of COVID-19, said Berger (Figure 6-3). Individual factors such as substance use or baseline health issues are exacerbated by existing health inequities, structural injustice, structural racism, and epistemic injustice. For immigrants and other marginalized populations, said Berger, COVID-19 *is* Long COVID, saying "We are dealing with a slow-moving, multidimensional, multidomain social catastrophe." *All* of these issues need to be addressed by primary care providers, advocates, patients, caregivers, and residents of the United States.

Berger offered suggestions on what needs to be done to address Long COVID on a number of levels. First, clinicians need to evaluate each patient holistically, and to reduce harm to patients while validating, assessing, and documenting their experiences. In addition, clinicians need to recognize the challenges of epistemic injustices and the harms caused to vulnerable populations. Berger explained that epistemic injustice can occur when patients are not listened to, are misdiagnosed, or are mismanaged; this is a phenomenon that patients and caregivers are "all too familiar with," particularly in chronic and poorly understood conditions such as Long COVID. Clinicians need to acknowledge the bias, stigma, fears, and assumptions that surround Long COVID, and discuss how our systems exacerbate health care barriers and perpetuate intersectional injustices. Clinicians should not limit themselves to the individual or biomedical domain, said Berger, but should work to reduce inequities by, for example, advocating for eviction moratoriums, providing economic support for workers, providing language concordant care, and decarcerating. In short, said Berger, "We need to empower and emphasize structural equity and epistemic humility." We need solidarity between health care workers and patients, we need to empower patients to take control, and we need to listen to those with Long COVID about their experiences, he concluded.

Berger summarized his main ideas:

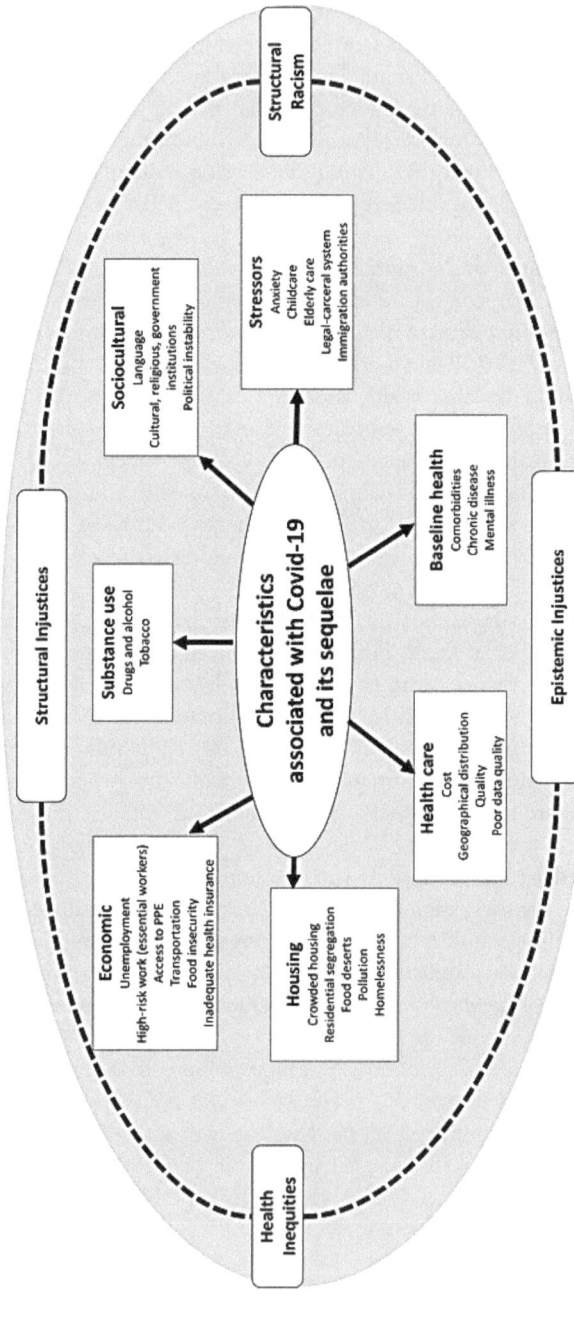

FIGURE 6-3 Characteristics associated with COVID-19 and Long COVID.
SOURCE: Republished with permission of John Wiley & Sons, from Berger et al., 2021, p. 523, in Zackary Berger presentation, March 22, 2022.

- COVID-19 and its long-term sequelae are strongly influenced by social determinants such as poverty and by structural inequalities such as racism and discrimination.
- Primary care providers are in a unique position to provide and coordinate care for vulnerable patients with Long COVID.
- Potential policy measures include strengthening primary care, optimizing data quality, and addressing the multiple nested domains of inequity.

DISCUSSION

Following the presentations, Verduzco-Gutierrez moderated a question-and-answer session, posing questions from planning committee members, representatives from SSA, and other workshop participants.

What is the role of telemedicine in Long COVID care, particularly for mental health issues?

Telehealth visits can be a great initial screening tool, said Abramoff, and are used by many if not most Long COVID clinics for the initial evaluation. Telehealth can be an effective way to connect with patients who may fatigue easily or have difficulty getting to an appointment, as well as patients who do not live in an area with a Long COVID clinic. Of course, he said, in-person follow-up is necessary to maximize outcomes and do further assessment.

What types of structured tests or assessments are useful for evaluating patients with Long COVID?

Some standardized tests may be useful for certain patients and clinicians, said Berger. However, he said that he worries about "the potential for ruling people in or out of having Long COVID on the basis of a structured instrument." This happens a lot in other chronic conditions such as depression or fibromyalgia, he said, with patients being "ruled out" if they do not meet certain criteria. Verduzco-Gutierrez added that another risk of structured instruments is that people may be "ruled in" for a condition because of symptoms that are related but not the same. For example, she said, a Long COVID patient may indicate that they have trouble concentrating on a depression questionnaire, but their inability to concentrate is caused by brain fog rather than depression.

Are there any national efforts to capture patients who traditionally fall through the cracks and may not have access to care for COVID-19 or Long COVID?

Since the start of the pandemic, said Berger, there has been heterogeneity and insufficient data gathering on vulnerable populations. The COVID

Tracking Project was developed in an attempt to gather data that the CDC was not, but there is still a lack of data on populations such as LGBTQ individuals or people who speak a language other than English. "We are not where we should be" regarding collecting data for vulnerable communities, he said. Berger added that there have been recommendations that a standing group of health care workers undertake a survey of populations affected by COVID-19. This would be a combination of a work program and a health census program, he said. Much of the research that has been conducted on COVID-19 has been done via the Internet or phone, which misses a lot of people. "If we really want to find people that are not being found," he said, "we need to go to where they are."

Further, he said, we need equal access to care in the broadest sense. Just being able to walk in the door of a clinic does not guarantee equal care, because inequities persist even with equal access. Verduzco-Gutierrez added that there is a need for policy to ensure that multidisciplinary clinics are able to care for all the patients who need it, regardless of ability to pay or insurance coverage. She added that some patients may not be eligible for care at a clinic because they were not able to access a test to document their COVID-19 infection. This phenomenon exacerbates the existing inequities in access.

How can primary care providers be supported in screening for and recognizing Long COVID?

The guidance statements from AAPM&R are designed to address the questions that primary care providers may have about symptoms, said Abramoff. There are efforts to take these statements and make them easier to use by primary providers by creating infographics, evaluation templates, and other tools. The effort to put the necessary information in the hands of clinicians across the country is ongoing, he said. Morrow added that the pediatric guidance that will be coming out soon is designed to be helpful for primary care pediatricians; it is symptom based but includes guidance on initial workup and treatment recommendations.

How are integrated specialty clinics measuring the effectiveness of their work?

This is a challenge, said Abramoff. Many clinics use their own measurement tools that were developed at the beginning of the pandemic. There are efforts to standardize tools, but these efforts take time. Verduzco-Gutierrez added that the demand for care is so high in some clinics that it can be difficult to get patients back in to see if things are working.

What are the challenges in differentiating the effect of COVID-19 infection from the effect of the pandemic in general in pediatric populations, particularly in terms of developmental and cognitive delay?

The pandemic and associated school closures have definitely had an impact on kids' mental health and overall well-being, said Morrow. Neuropsychology testing that looks at specific cognitive constructs has found issues with attention in some Long COVID patients; this is less likely to be a pandemic effect, particularly when we control for mood symptoms. However, the effect of the pandemic in general is "something we are always thinking about."

Are children with Long COVID getting the accommodations they need in schools? As they get these accommodations, will that potentially help other students with disabilities that are not related to COVID-19?

Simply increasing awareness of Long COVID and how an illness can affect overall function and ability to participate in school can be helpful, said Morrow, and this awareness can carry over to other conditions as well. Establishing protocols for accommodations for students with Long COVID certainly has the potential to help others.

What has been the experience of clinics that help patients with disability paperwork? Do patients tend to get denied or get approved?

Abramoff said that the patients at his clinic tend to get covered but it is challenging, with multiple rounds of back and forth. He said that the process wears down some patients and they "stop fighting after a while" because of the enormous burden of filling out paperwork and updating it regularly. Every employer and insurance company weighs different information, and it can be challenging for a provider to give information in the way that is most supportive of the patient. Berger added that some patients fall through the cracks because they simply do not have the energy or resources to keep filling out the forms. "It takes energy to be the squeaky wheel," he said, and many patients do not have the time to continue the fight. Verduzco-Gutierrez agreed that the process is overwhelming, and she added that some disability insurance companies deny patients because the companies do not take into account symptoms like postexertional malaise or the unseen fatigue that follows cognitive work.

7

Exploring Future Directions in the Treatment of Long COVID

Developing vaccines and therapeutics for acute COVID-19 infection within a year of the epidemic was one of the "greatest achievements of medicine in the past few decades," said Steven Deeks, professor of medicine in residence at the University of California, San Francisco. However, it was "pretty straightforward" because the virus was easy to target for vaccines, the targets for therapeutics were well-characterized, and regulators and industry leaders were motivated to work quickly and efficiently. Unfortunately, "none of this really applies" to the treatment of Long COVID, said Deeks.

Deeks identified a number of challenges confronting the development of effective treatments for Long COVID. There are several distinct phenotypes of Long COVID, in which symptoms are focused on the cardiovascular, pulmonary, or neurocognitive systems. Long COVID involves multiple mechanisms, including direct irreversible tissue injury, inflammation, autoantibodies, and microvascular clotting. There are multiple effects on the body such as nerve damage or organ damage, and multiple types of outcomes, including postural orthostatic tachycardia syndrome (POTS), myalgic encephalomyelitis/chronic fatigue syndrome (ME/CFS), and mast cell activation syndrome (MCAS). People are at increased susceptibility to COVID-19 and Long COVID for a huge variety of reasons, including socioeconomic factors, preexisting conditions, mental health history, sex, race, age, and access to health care. Further, said Deeks, there is not a thorough understanding of the natural history of Long COVID, and symptoms within an individual can wax and wane. Developing treatments—and developing ways to measure whether these treatments are effective—is enormously challenging because of all of this variation.

Deeks described the current approach to the management of Long COVID. The Centers for Disease Control and Prevention (CDC) says that Long COVID can be diagnosed and managed by primary care, and suggests a conservative approach for the first 4 to 12 weeks, with an aggressive workup at 12 weeks if symptoms persist (CDC, 2021a). A variety of physical tests may be employed, including orthostatic vital signs, ambulatory pulse, and exercise capacity. Laboratory testing can be conducted in order to confirm previous COVID-19 infection and to rule out common conditions with similar symptoms (e.g., arthritis, thyroid issues). Specialized testing for Long COVID may include the tilt test, a chest CT, or a brain MRI. Deeks warned that excessive testing can be harmful, as it can lead "down various rabbit holes." Another issue with testing, he said, can be if a patient's subjective experience does not align with the objective findings.

The goal of Long COVID treatment is to improve the patient's quality of life, and a holistic approach is helpful for meeting this aim, observed Deeks. He listed some of the commonly used therapies, including compression stockings, physical therapy, pacing of activities, flexibility and strength exercises, and medications. There are medications for specific diagnoses (e.g., selective serotonin reuptake inhibitors for depression), and some clinicians prescribe other medications off-label (e.g., antivirals, intravenous immunoglobulin). Deeks said that a multidisciplinary, team-based approach for treatment is critical, as it can simultaneously address physical issues, mental health issues, social support, and rehabilitation. In addition, these types of clinics can validate the experiences of patients, help them cope with uncertainty, and help them access financial and other types of support.

Deeks said a search on ClinicalTrials.gov listed over 90 interventional studies related to Long COVID,[1] including studies on drugs, biologics, rehabilitation interventions, medical devices, and complementary and alternative therapies. He said that, novel research designs, such as adaptive platform trials, are likely to emerge in the area of Long COVID treatment, much as they did for the management of acute COVID-19 infection.

Because multiple pathways are involved in the development of Long COVID, said Deeks, it is possible that multiple types of interventions may be necessary. For example, if the virus causes irreversible tissue damage, physical therapy and rehabilitation are more likely to benefit the patient. If the patient's symptoms are caused by the virus persisting in the body, therapeutic

---

[1] ClinicalTrials.gov is a resource provided by the U.S. National Library of Medicine: https://clinicaltrials.gov (accessed March 21, 2022).

vaccinations may be of use. Anti-inflammatory drugs and anticoagulants could address specific issues within the body. Antiviral therapies may not only be useful in preventing Long COVID, they may be useful in the chronic setting as well.

Many studies focus on quality of life and functional status as the outcomes of interest, he said, which poses regulatory challenges. Multiple biologic mechanisms and hard-to-define clinical outcomes that wax and wane will make drug development challenging. Further, limited industry engagement remains a major barrier, said Deeks. Despite these challenges, targetable pathways have been identified and proof-of-concept studies are underway, which can help us understand the biology behind Long COVID as well as identify potential therapies.

DISCUSSION

Following Deeks' presentation, Andrea Lerner, physician and medical officer at the National Institute of Allergy and Infectious Diseases of the NIH, facilitated a panel discussion with Deeks, Frontera, and Nath, taking questions from the workshop participants.

Given that the majority of Long COVID cases develop in people with mild symptoms who receive no intervention, could COVID-19 treatments given at the outset of a positive COVID-19 case eliminate or significantly reduce the incidence of Long COVID?

Deeks replied that while there is no evidence in this area, it "makes sense" that the earlier therapy is started, the better the outcomes will be. For almost any infectious disease, such as HIV, early therapy is beneficial.

Are there specific symptoms of Long COVID that have shown response to physical therapy, or is the benefit of therapy limited until the cause of the symptoms has been resolved?

In the acute phase of COVID-19, early rehabilitation has been shown to have beneficial effects, including shortening length of stay and enhancing pulmonary recovery, said Frontera. In Long COVID, evidence is limited, but there are good indications that symptoms such as shortness of breath and fatigue respond well to exercise interventions. The results are consistent among the small number of studies (Foged et al., 2021; Wasilewski et al., 2022) that have been conducted in this area, he said, but we will need to follow patients for a longer period of time to determine if therapy has been curative.

Given that specialty clinics and centers of excellence may disproportionately treat primarily White, more financially secure patients, how can we prevent these centers from exacerbating disparities?

There was great progress made in securing access to HIV care for lower-income and marginalized populations, said Deeks. This was accomplished through massive investment from the federal government; this investment means that patients, regardless of financial means or insurance, can go to clinics and receive primary care, specialty care, social services, psychiatric care, and so on. Deeks said there is some discussion in California to fund this type of approach for Long COVID. He added that while it will be an expensive endeavor to provide this holistic approach, right now, "people have no options." Frontera said that the issue of access and disparities is common in the field of rehabilitation because most centers that treat complex conditions are located in academic medical centers. One option, he said, is to develop a specialized clinic and then make it available to smaller hospitals via telehealth. The effectiveness of this approach is under investigation, he said, but it could be one that works for improving access to care for Long COVID.

How do we strike the balance between the need to start trials to find effective therapeutics for Long COVID and the need to understand different phenotypes and subtypes of post-COVID conditions so trial populations are not so heterogenous that any effect is masked?

It is not easy, said Nath. Studies need carefully characterized inclusion criteria, which generally results in small sample sizes. However, if a study uses a larger, heterogeneous population, "you will never find anything." Nath shared an example of a study he and his colleagues conducted for chronic fatigue syndrome. Out of an initial group of 250 patients, 21 were enrolled, all of whom had an infection before they developed symptoms, and all of whom had the same pattern of symptoms. A study like this will by its nature examine a narrow population that may not be at all generalizable for the general population. Deeks added that these types of studies can also help further our understanding of biology, mechanisms, and clinical phenotypes. Nath agreed and said that in the study that narrowed to 21 patients, data were collected on all 250 initial patients, which helped further the understanding of the condition. Nath said that another illustrative example of this tension can be seen in studies on postinfectious syndromes. For example, herpes encephalitis is an antibody-mediated phenomenon, so therapies include intravenous immunoglobulin or anti-B cell therapies. Other kinds of postinfectious syndromes, such as acute disseminated encephalomyelitis, are a T-cell-mediated phenomenon, so the treatment would be very different. With Long COVID, said Nath, we may find that even the immunotypic profile of post-COVID-19 patients is heterogeneous.

Is there any evidence that specific variants of COVID-19 affect the development of Long COVID differently?

Anecdotally, said Deeks, the worst cases of Long COVID are from the first couple of waves. However, it is a complicated question because variants occurred in different eras of the pandemic. For example, Delta happened in an era when there were vaccines and treatments emerging. Deeks said he is not aware of any good data on this question. Probably the most important question, he said, is whether and to what extent the Omicron variant causes Long COVID. The numbers of people who have been infected with Omicron is so massive, both in the United States and globally, that if the frequency of Long COVID is the same as with previous variants, "we are going to be in big trouble." There will be a massive wave of people with really serious issues, he said, that will overwhelm primary care physicians, primary care clinics, and Long COVID clinics.

What are meaningful clinical trial outcomes for Long COVID therapeutics?

The endpoints in our studies are subjective, said Nath, and "that is the biggest problem." There are well-accepted scales, such as the Health Utility Index, that are validated, but they are still subjective. Taking this type of evidence to the U.S. Food and Drug Administration (FDA) for drug approval could be challenging, he said, although FDA does have experience with treating pain and depression and other conditions that include subjective measures. Frontera added that there are several outcomes that are important for Long COVID, including fatigue and intolerance to exercise. For the purposes of determining if a person could perform work, it could be useful to look separately at cardiovascular tolerance and neuromuscular tolerance. The specific testing that is useful depends on the nature of the job activity, he said.

How can patients educate doctors who do not understand the experience of Long COVID?

One approach that has been useful in the world of rehabilitation, said Frontera, is to invite patients to talk to residents in training about their personal experience with different conditions. This has been helpful for doctors to understand conditions such as amputations and traumatic brain injury, and may be useful in Long COVID as well.

When will a therapeutic for Long COVID become available?

This will likely take time, said Deeks, but much progress is being made. We are making progress on identifying the mechanisms of Long COVID, particularly how inflammation can result in a number of outcomes. Once the mechanisms are clearly identified, there will be advances that can be made and clinical trials can be started.

Is it possible that what is now known as PASC will eventually be categorized as several different conditions, based on the mechanism or end effect?

Deeks responded that this is already the case in some ways. Some conditions that are associated with Long COVID have been identified and have different mechanisms and therapies, for example, post-ICU syndrome and POTS.

CLOSE OF WORKSHOP

At the close of the workshop, Frontera thanked SSA for its support; thanked the speakers for sharing their knowledge, expertise, experience, and ideas; and thanked the workshop participants for their many thought-provoking comments and questions. Frontera adjourned the workshop.

Appendix A

References

Abdel-Mannan, O., M. Eyre, U. Löbel, A. Bamford, C. Eltze, B. Hameed, C. Hemingway, and Y. Hacohen. 2020. Neurologic and radiographic findings associated with COVID-19 infection in children. *JAMA Neurology* 77(11):1440. https://dx.doi.org/10.1001/jamaneurol.2020.2687 (accessed June 14, 2022).

American Academy of Pediatrics. 2022. *Children and COVID-19: State-level data report.* https://www.aap.org/en/pages/2019-novel-coronavirus-covid-19-infections/children-and-covid-19-state-level-data-report/ (accessed May 11, 2022).

American Academy of Physical Medicine and Rehabilitation. 2022. *PASC dashboard.* https://pascdashboard.aapmr.org/ (accessed May 12, 2022).

Arroll, B., F. Goodyear-Smith, S. Crengle, J. Gunn, N. Kerse, T. Fishman, K. Falloon, and S. Hatcher. 2010. Validation of PHQ-2 and PHQ-9 to screen for major depression in the primary care population. *Annals of Family Medicine* 8(4):348-353. https://doi.org/10.1370/afm.1139.

Ayoubkhani, D., P. Pawelek, and M. Bosworth. 2021. *Prevalence of ongoing symptoms following coronavirus (COVID-19) infection in the UK: 5 August 2021.* https://www.ons.gov.uk/peoplepopulationandcommunity/healthandsocialcare/conditionsanddiseases/bulletins/prevalenceofongoingsymptomsfollowingcoronaviruscovid19infectionintheuk/5august2021 (accessed June 17, 2022).

Balcom, E. F., A. Nath, and C. Power. 2021. Acute and chronic neurological disorders in COVID-19: Potential mechanisms of disease. *Brain* 144(12):3576-3588. https://dx.doi.org/10.1093/brain/awab302.

Beauchamp, M. K., D. Joshi, J. McMillan, U. Erbas Oz, L. E. Griffith, N. E. Basta, S. Kirkland, C. Wolfson, P. Raina, A. Costa, L. Anderson, C. Balion, A. Yukiko, B. Cossette, M. Levasseur, S. Hofer, T. Paterson, D. Hogan, T. Liu-Ambrose, V. Menec, P. St. John, G. Mugford, Z. Gao, V. Taler, P. Davidson, A. Wister, and T. Cosco. 2022. Assessment of functional mobility after COVID-19 in adults aged 50 years or older in the Canadian Longitudinal Study on Aging. *JAMA Network Open* 5(1):e2146168. https://dx.doi.org/10.1001/jamanetworkopen.2021.46168.

Beck, A. T., R. A. Steer, and M. G. Carbin. 1988. Psychometric properties of the Beck Depression Inventory: Twenty-five years of evaluation. *Clinical Psychology Review* 8(1):77-100. https://doi.org/10.1016/0272-7358(88)90050-5.

Becker, C., K. Beck, S. Zumbrunn, V. Memma, N. Herzog, B. Bissmann, S. Gross, N. Loretz, J. Mueller, S. A. Amacher, C. Bohren, R. Schaefert, S. Bassetti, C. Fux, B. Mueller, P. Schuetz, and S. Hunziker. 2021. Long COVID 1 year after hospitalisation for COVID-19: A prospective bicentric cohort study. *Swiss Medical Weekly* 151:w30091. https://doi.org/10.4414/smw.2021.w30091.

Bek, L. M., J. C. Berentschot, M. E. Hellemons, S. M. Huijts, J. G. J. V. Aerts, J. van Bommel, M. E. van Genderen, D. A. M. P. J. Gommers, G. M. Ribbers, M. H. Heijenbrok-Kal, R. J. G. van den Berg-Emons, and the CO-FLOW Collaboration Group. 2021. CO-FLOW: COVID-19 follow-up care paths and long-term outcomes within the Dutch health care system: Study protocol of a multicenter prospective cohort study following patients 2 years after hospital discharge. *BMC Health Services Research* 21(1):847. https://doi.org/10.1186/s12913-021-06813-6.

Bell, D. S., K. Jordan, and M. Robinson. 2001. Thirteen-year follow-up of children and adolescents with chronic fatigue syndrome. *Pediatrics* 107(5):994-998. https://dx.doi.org/10.1542/peds.107.5.994.

Berger, Z., V. Altiery de Jesus, S. A. Assoumou, and T. Greenhalgh. 2021. Long COVID and health inequities: The role of primary care. *Milbank Quarterly* 99(2):519-541. https://doi.org/10.1111/1468-0009.12505.

Boldrini, M., P. D. Canoll, and R. S. Klein. 2021. How COVID-19 affects the brain. *JAMA Psychiatry* 78(6):682. https://dx.doi.org/10.1001/jamapsychiatry.2021.0500.

Borch, L., M. Holm, M. Knudsen, S. Ellermann-Eriksen, and S. Hagstroem. 2022. Long COVID symptoms and duration in SARS-CoV-2 positive children—a nationwide cohort study. *European Journal of Pediatrics* 181(4):1597-1607. https://dx.doi.org/10.1007/s00431-021-04345-z.

Brackel, C., L. Noij, C. L. Legghe, S. Vijverberg, S. Hashimoto, A. H. Maitland-van der Zee, D. Munblit, T. Stephenson D. Buonsenso, M. Ryd-Rinder, D. W. Miller, A. M. Edwards, M. McVoy, and S. W. J. Terheggen. 2022. *Uniting global efforts on pediatric Long-COVID: Results of the International Pediatric Post-COVID Condition in Children Collaboration (IP4C)*. https://doi.org/10.1164/ajrccm-conference.2022.205.1_MeetingAbstracts.A1157.

Buonsenso, D., D. Munblit, C. De Rose, D. Sinatti, A. Ricchiuto, A. Carfi, and P. Valentini. 2021. Preliminary evidence on long COVID in children. *Acta Paediatrica* 110(7):2208-2211. https://dx.doi.org/10.1111/apa.15870.

CDC (Centers for Disease Control and Prevention). 2021a. *General clinical considerations: Evaluating and caring for patients with post-COVID conditions: Interim guidance.* https://www.cdc.gov/coronavirus/2019-ncov/hcp/clinical-care/post-covid-clinical-eval.html (accessed May 11, 2022).

CDC. 2021b. *Interim guidance on evaluating and caring for patients with post-COVID conditions.* https://www.cdc.gov/coronavirus/2019-ncov/hcp/clinical-care/post-covid-index.html (accessed May 11, 2022).

Chen, C., S. R. Haupert, L. Zimmermann, X. Shi, L. G. Fritsche, and B. Mukherjee. 2022. Global prevalence of post COVID-19 condition or long COVID: A meta-analysis and systematic review. *Journal of Infectious Diseases.* https://dx.doi.org/10.1093/infdis/jiac136.

Cirulli, E. T., K. M. Schiabor Barrett, S. Riffle, A. Bolze, I. Neveux, S. Dabe, J. J. Grzymski, J. T. Lu, and N. L. Washington. 2020. Long-term COVID-19 symptoms in a large unselected population. MedRxiv. https://doi.org/10.1101/2020.10.07.20208702.

Clarke, K. E., J. M. Jones, Y. Deng, E. Nycz, A. Lee, R. Iachan, A. V. Gundlapalli, A. J. Hall, and A. MacNeil. 2022. Seroprevalence of infection-induced SARS-CoV-2 antibodies — United States, September 2021–February 2022. *Morbidity and Mortality Weekly Report* 71(17):606-608. http://dx.doi.org/10.15585/mmwr.mm7117e3.

Crook, H., S. Raza, J. Nowell, M. Young, and P. Edison. 2021. Long COVID—mechanisms, risk factors, and management. *BMJ.* https://dx.doi.org/10.1136/bmj.n1648.

Derose, K. P., J. J. Escarce, and N. Lurie. 2007. Immigrants and health care: Sources of vulnerability. *Health Affairs* 26(5):1258-1268. https://doi.org/10.1377/hlthaff.26.5.1258.

Dias, F. A., A. L. N. Cunha, P. M. P. Pantoja, C. L. Moreira, P. J. Tomaselli, M. C. Zanon Zotin, F. A. Colleto, S. R. Cabette Fabio, O. M. Pontes-Neto, and W. Marques Júnior. 2021. Acute inflammatory painful polyradiculoneuritis. *Neurology: Clinical Practice* 11(2):e205-e207. https://dx.doi.org/10.1212/cpj.0000000000000910.

Dundumalla, S., S. Barshikar, W. N. Niehaus, A. F. Ambrose, S. Y. Kim, and B. A. Abramoff. 2022. A survey of dedicated PASC clinics: Characteristics, barriers and spirit of collaboration. *PM&R* 14(3):348-356. https://doi.org/10.1002/pmrj.12766.

Ekbom, E., R. Frithiof, E. Öi, I. M. Larson, M. Lipcsey, S. Rubertsson, E. Wallin, C. Janson, M. Hultström, and A. Malinovschi. 2021. Impaired diffusing capacity for carbon monoxide is common in critically ill COVID-19 patients at four months post-discharge. *Respiratory Medicine* 182:106394. https://doi.org/10.1016/j.rmed.2021.106394.

EuroQoL Research Foundation. n.d. *Home page.* https://euroqol.org/ (accessed May 11, 2022).

Foged, F., I. E. Rasmussen, J. Bjørn Budde, R. S. Rasmussen, V. Rasmussen, M. Lyngbæk, S. Jønck, R. Krogh-Madsen, B. Lindegaard, M. Ried-Larsen, R. M. G. Berg, and R. H. Christensen. 2021. Fidelity, tolerability and safety of acute high-intensity interval training after hospitalisation for COVID-19: A randomised cross-over trial. *BMJ Open Sport & Exercise Medicine* 7(3):e001156. https://doi.org/10.1136/bmjsem-2021-001156.

Frontera, W., F. Gimigliano, J. Melvin, J. Li, L. Li, J. Lains, and G. Stucki. 2019. ClinFIT: ISPRM's universal functioning information tool based on the WHO's ICF. *Journal of the International Society of Physical and Rehabilitation Medicine* 2(1):19-21. https://doi.org/10.4103/jisprm.jisprm_36_19.

García-Abellán, J., S. Padilla, M. Fernández-González, J. A. García, V. Agulló, M. Andreo, S. Ruiz, A. Galiana, F. Gutiérrez, and M. Masiá. 2021. Antibody response to SARS-CoV-2 is associated with long-term clinical outcome in patients with COVID-19: A longitudinal study. *Journal of Clinical Immunology* 41(7):1490-1501. https://doi.org/10.1007/s10875-021-01083-7.

George, P. M., S. L. Barratt, R. Condliffe, S. R. Desai, A. Devaraj, I. Forrest, M. A. Gibbons, N. Hart, R. G. Jenkins, D. F. McAuley, B. V. Patel, E. Thwaite, and L. G. Spencer. 2020. Respiratory follow-up of patients with COVID-19 pneumonia. *Thorax* 75(11):1009-1016. https://dx.doi.org/10.1136/thoraxjnl-2020-215314.

González-Hermosillo, J. A., J. P. Martínez-López, S. A. Carrillo-Lampón, D. Ruiz-Ojeda, S. Herrera-Ramírez, L. M. Amezcua-Guerra, and M. D. R. Martínez-Alvarado. 2021. Post-acute COVID-19 symptoms, a potential link with myalgic encephalomyelitis/chronic fatigue syndrome: A 6-month survey in a Mexican cohort. *Brain Sciences* 11(6):760. https://dx.doi.org/10.3390/brainsci11060760.

Groff, D., A. Sun, A. E. Ssentongo, D. M. Ba, N. Parsons, G. R. Poudel, A. Lekoubou, J. S. Oh, J. E. Ericson, P. Ssentongo, and V. M. Chinchilli. 2021. Short-term and long-term rates of postacute sequelae of SARS-CoV-2 infection. *JAMA Network Open* 4(10):e2128568. https://dx.doi.org/10.1001/jamanetworkopen.2021.28568.

Hanson, S. W., C. Abbafati, J. G. Aerts, Z. Al-Aly, C. Ashbaugh, T. Ballouz, O. Blyuss, P. Bobkova, G. Bonsel, S. Borzakova, D. Buonsenso, D. Butnaru, A. Carter, H. Chu, C. De Rose, M. M. Diab, E. Ekbom, M. El Tantawi, V. Fomin, R. Frithiof, A. Gamirova, P. V. Glybochko, J. A. Haagsma, S. H. Javanmard, E. B. Hamilton, G. Harris, M. H. Heijenbrok-Kal, R. Helbok, M. E. Hellemons, D. Hillus, S. M. Huijts, M. Hultström, W. Jassat, F. Kurth, I.-M. Larsson, M. Lipcsey, C. Liu, C. D. Loflin, A. Malinovschi, W. Mao, L. Mazankova, D. McCulloch, D. Menges, N. Mohammadifard, D. Munblit, N. A. Nekliudov, O. Ogbuoji, I. M. Osmanov, J. L. Peñalvo, M. S. Petersen, M. A. Puhan, M. Rahman, V. Rass, N. Reinig, G. M. Ribbers, A. Ricchiuto, S. Rubertsson, E. Samitova, N. Sarrafzadegan, A. Shikhaleva, K. E. Simpson, D. Sinatti, J. B. Soriano, E. Spiridonova, F. Steinbeis, A. A. Svistunov, P. Valentini, B. J. Van De Water, R. Van Den Berg-Emons, E. Wallin, M. Witzenrath, Y. Wu, H. Xu, T. Zoller, C. Adolph, J. Albright, J. O. Amlag, A. Y. Aravkin, B. L. Bang-Jensen, C. Bisignano, R. Castellano, E. Castro, S. Chakrabarti, J. K. Collins, X. Dai, F. Daoud, C. Dapper, A. Deen, B. B. Duncan, M. Erickson, S. B. Ewald, A. J. Ferrari, A. D. Flaxman, N. Fullman, A. Gamkrelidze, J. R. Giles, G. Guo, S. I. Hay, J. He, M. Helak, E. N. Hulland, M. Kereselidze, K. J. Krohn, A. Lazzar-Atwood, A. Lindstrom, R. Lozano, B. Magistro, D. C. Malta, J. Månsson, A. M. Mantilla Herrera, A. H. Mokdad, L. Monasta, S. Nomura, M. Pasovic, D. M. Pigott, R. C. Reiner, G. Reinke, A. L. P. Ribeiro, D. F. Santomauro, A. Sholokhov, E. E. Spurlock, R. Walcott, A. Walker, C. S. Wiysonge, P. Zheng, J. P. Bettger, C. J. Murray, and T. Vos. 2022. *A global systematic analysis of the occurrence, severity, and recovery pattern of long COVID in 2020 and 2021.* MedRxiv. https://doi.org/10.1101/2022.05.26.22275532.

Haute Autorité de Santé, France. 2021. *Covid long: Les recommandations de la Haute Autorité de Santé.* https://www.service-public.fr/particuliers/actualites/A14678?lang=en (accessed May 31, 2022).

HealthMeasures. n.d. *Neuro-QoL Score Cut Points.* https://www.healthmeasures.net/score-and-interpret/interpret-scores/neuro-qol/neuro-qol-score-cut-points (accessed June 10, 2022).

Herdman, M., C. Gudex, A. Lloyd, M. Janssen, P. Kind, D. Parkin, G. Bonsel, and X. Badia. 2011. Development and preliminary testing of the new five-level version of EQ-5D (EQ-5D-5L). *Quality of Life Research* 20(10):1727-1736. https://dx.doi.org/10.1007/s11136-011-9903-x.

Hernández-Ronquillo, L., F. Moien-Afshari, K. Knox, J. Britz, and J. F. Téllez-Zenteno. 2011. How to measure fatigue in epilepsy? The validation of three scales for clinical use. *Epilepsy Research* 95(1):119-129. https://www.sciencedirect.com/science/article/pii/S0920121111000787/ (accessed June 15, 2022).

Herridge, M. S., A. M. Cheung, C. M. Tansey, A. Matte-Martyn, N. Diaz-Granados, F. Al-Saidi, A. B. Cooper, C. B. Guest, C. D. Mazer, S. Mehta, T. E. Stewart, A. Barr, D. Cook, and A. S. Slutsky. 2003. One-year outcomes in survivors of the acute respiratory distress syndrome. *New England Journal of Medicine* 348(8):683-693. https://dx.doi.org/10.1056/nejmoa022450.

Huang, C., L. Huang, Y. Wang, X. Li, L. Ren, X. Gu, L. Kang, L. Guo, M. Liu, X. Zhou, J. Luo, Z. Huang, S. Tu, Y. Zhao, L. Chen, D. Xu, Y. Li, C. Li, L. Peng, Y. Li, W. Xie, D. Cui, L. Shang, G. Fan, J. Xu, G. Wang, Y. Wang, J. Zhong, C. Wang, J. Wang, D. Zhang, and B. Cao. 2021a. 6-month consequences of COVID-19 in patients discharged from hospital: A cohort study. *Lancet* 397(10270):220-232. https://dx.doi.org/10.1016/s0140-6736(20)32656-8.

Huang, L., Q. Yao, X. Gu, Q. Wang, L. Ren, Y. Wang, P. Hu, L. Guo, M. Liu, J. Xu, X. Zhang, Y. Qu, Y. Fan, X. Li, C. Li, T. Yu, J. Xia, M. Wei, L. Chen, Y. Li, F. Xiao, D. Liu, J. Wang, X. Wang, and B. Cao. 2021b. 1-year outcomes in hospital survivors with COVID-19: A longitudinal cohort study. *Lancet* 398(10302):747-758. https://dx.doi.org/10.1016/s0140-6736(21)01755-4.

Hultström, M., R. Frithiof, M. Lipcsey, S. Rubertsson, E. Wallin, and I.-M. Larsson. 2021. *Follow-up of critical COVID-19 patients (FUP-COVID).* https://clinicaltrials.gov/ct2/show/NCT04474249 (accessed June 17, 2022).

IOM (Institute of Medicine). 2015. *Beyond myalgic encephalomyelitis/chronic fatigue syndrome: Redefining an illness.* Washington, DC: The National Academies Press. https://doi.org/10.17226/19012.

Iverson, G. L., E. J. Connors, J. Marsh, and D. P. Terry. 2021. Examining normative reference values and item-level symptom endorsement for the quality of life in neurological disorders (Neuro-QoL) v2.0 Cognitive Function-Short Form. *Archives of Clinical Neuropsychology* 36(1):126-134. https://dx.doi.org/10.1093/arclin/acaa044.

Johns, M. W. 1991. A new method for measuring daytime sleepiness: The Epworth Sleepiness Scale. *Sleep* 14(6):540-545. https://doi.org/10.1093/sleep/14.6.540.

Kikkenborg Berg, S., S. Dam Nielsen, U. Nygaard, H. Bundgaard, P. Palm, C. Rotvig, and A. Vinggaard Christensen. 2022. Long COVID symptoms in SARS-CoV-2-positive adolescents and matched controls (LongCovidKidsDK): A national, cross-sectional study. *Lancet Child and Adolescent Health* 6(4):240-248. https://doi.org/10.1016/s2352-4642(22)00004-9.

Kroenke, K., R. L. Spitzer, and J. B. W. Williams. 2003. The Patient Health Questionnaire-2: Validity of a two-item depression screener. *Medical Care* 41(11). https://doi.org/10.1097/01.MLR.0000093487.78664.3C.

Learmonth, Y. C., D. Dlugonski, L. A. Pilutti, B. M. Sandroff, R. Klaren, and R. W. Motl. 2013. Psychometric properties of the Fatigue Severity Scale and the Modified Fatigue Impact Scale. *Journal of the Neurological Sciences* 331(1):102-107. https://doi.org/10.1016/j.jns.2013.05.023.

Lee, J., S. D. Vernon, P. Jeys, W. Ali, A. Campos, D. Unutmaz, B. Yellman, and L. Bateman. 2020. Hemodynamics during the 10-minute NASA Lean Test: Evidence of circulatory decompensation in a subset of ME/CFS patients. *Journal of Translational Medicine* 18(1):314. https://doi.org/10.1186/s12967-020-02481-y.

Lee, M.-H., D. P. Perl, G. Nair, W. Li, D. Maric, H. Murray, S. J. Dodd, A. P. Koretsky, J. A. Watts, V. Cheung, E. Masliah, I. Horkayne-Szakaly, R. Jones, M. N. Stram, J. Moncur, M. Hefti, R. D. Folkerth, and A. Nath. 2021. Microvascular injury in the brains of patients with Covid-19. *New England Journal of Medicine* 384(5):481-483. https://dx.doi.org/10.1056/nejmc2033369.

Lerdal, A., and A. Kottorp. 2011. Psychometric properties of the Fatigue Severity Scale—Rasch analyses of individual responses in a Norwegian stroke cohort. *International Journal of Nursing Studies* 48(10):1258-1265. https://doi.org/10.1016/j.ijnurstu.2011.02.019.

Lopez-Leon, S., T. Wegman-Ostrosky, C. Perelman, R. Sepulveda, P. A. Rebolledo, A. Cuapio, and S. Villapol. 2021. More than 50 long-term effects of COVID-19: A systematic review and meta-analysis. *Scientific Reports* 11:16144. https://doi.org/10.1038/s41598-021-95565-8.

Ludvigsson, J. F. 2021. Case report and systematic review suggest that children may experience similar long-term effects to adults after clinical COVID-19. *Acta Paediatrica* 110(3):914-921. https://dx.doi.org/10.1111/apa.15673.

Mirfazeli, F. S., A. Sarabi-Jamab, V. Pereira-Sanchez, A. Kordi, B. Shariati, S. V. Shariat, S. Bahrami, S. Nohesara, M. Almasi-Dooghaee, and S. H. R. Faiz. 2022. Chronic fatigue syndrome and cognitive deficit are associated with acute-phase neuropsychiatric manifestations of COVID-19: A 9-month follow-up study. *Neurological Sciences* 43(4):2231-2239. https://dx.doi.org/10.1007/s10072-021-05786-y.

Molteni, E., C. H. Sudre, L. S. Canas, S. S. Bhopal, R. C. Hughes, M. Antonelli, B. Murray, K. Kläser, E. Kerfoot, L. Chen, J. Deng, C. Hu, S. Selvachandran, K. Read, J. Capdevila Pujol, A. Hammers, T. D. Spector, S. Ourselin, C. J. Steves, M. Modat, M. Absoud, and E. L. Duncan. 2021. Illness duration and symptom profile in symptomatic UK school-aged children tested for SARS-CoV-2. *Lancet Child and Adolescent Health* 5(10):708-718. https://dx.doi.org/10.1016/s2352-4642(21)00198-x.

Montani, D., L. Savale, N. Noel, O. Meyrignac, R. Colle, M. Gasnier, E. Corruble, A. Beurnier, E.-M. Jutant, T. Pham, A.-L. Lecoq, J.-F. Papon, S. Figueiredo, A. Harrois, M. Humbert, and X. Monnet. 2022. Post-acute COVID-19 syndrome. *European Respiratory Review* 31(163):210185. https://dx.doi.org/10.1183/16000617.0185-2021.

Munblit, D., P. Bobkova, E. Spiridonova, A. Shikhaleva, A. Gamirova, O. Blyuss, N. Nekliudov, P. Bugaeva, M. Andreeva, A. DunnGalvin, P. Comberiati, C. Apfelbacher, J. Genuneit, S. Avdeev, V. Kapustina, A. Guekht, V. Fomin, A. A. Svistunov, P. Timashev, V. S. Subbot, V. V. Royuk, T. M. Drake, S. W. Hanson, L. Merson, G. Carson, P. Horby, L. Sigfrid, J. T. Scott, M. G. Semple, J. O. Warner, T. Vos, P. Olliaro, P. Glybochko, and D. Butnaru. 2021. Incidence and risk factors for persistent symptoms in adults previously hospitalized for COVID-19. *Clinical and Experimental Allergy* 51(9):1107-1120. https://doi.org/10.1111/cea.13997.

Nalbandian, A., K. Sehgal, A. Gupta, M. V. Madhavan, C. McGroder, J. S. Stevens, J. R. Cook, A. S. Nordvig, D. Shalev, T. S. Sehrawat, N. Ahluwalia, B. Bikdeli, D. Dietz, C. Der-Nigoghossian, N. Liyanage-Don, G. F. Rosner, E. J. Bernstein, S. Mohan, A. A. Beckley, D. S. Seres, T. K. Choueiri, N. Uriel, J. C. Ausiello, D. Accili, D. E. Freedberg, M. Baldwin, A. Schwartz, D. Brodie, C. K. Garcia, M. S. V. Elkind, J. M. Connors, J. P. Bilezikian, D. W. Landry, and E. Y. Wan. 2021. Post-acute COVID-19 syndrome. *Nature Medicine* 27(4):601-615. https://dx.doi.org/10.1038/s41591-021-01283-z.

NICE (National Institute for Health and Care Excellence). 2020. COVID-19 rapid guideline: Managing the long-term effects of COVID-19. London, UK: National Institute for Health and Care Excellence. https://www.ncbi.nlm.nih.gov/books/NBK567261/ (accessed June 15, 2022).

Novak, P., S. S. Mukerji, H. S. Alabsi, D. Systrom, S. P. Marciano, D. Felsenstein, W. J. Mullally, and D. M. Pilgrim. 2022. Multisystem involvement in post-acute sequelae of coronavirus disease 19. *Annals of Neurology* 91(3):367-379. https://dx.doi.org/10.1002/ana.26286.

Novi, G., T. Rossi, E. Pedemonte, L. Saitta, C. Rolla, L. Roccatagliata, M. Inglese, and D. Farinini. 2020. Acute disseminated encephalomyelitis after SARS-CoV-2 infection. *Neurology: Neuroimmunology & Neuroinflammation* 7(5):e797. https://dx.doi.org/10.1212/nxi.0000000000000797.

Osmanov, I. M., E. Spiridonova, P. Bobkova, A. Gamirova, A. Shikhaleva, M. Andreeva, O. Blyuss, Y. El-Taravi, A. DunnGalvin, P. Comberiati, D. G. Peroni, C. Apfelbacher, J. Genuneit, L. Mazankova, A. Miroshina, E. Chistyakova, E. Samitova, S. Borzakova, E. Bondarenko, A. A. Korsunskiy, I. Konova, S. W. Hanson, G. Carson, L. Sigfrid, J. T. Scott, M. Greenhawt, E. A. Whittaker, E. Garralda, O. V. Swann, D. Buonsenso, D. E. Nicholls, F. Simpson, C. Jones, M. G. Semple, J. O. Warner, T. Vos, P. Olliaro, and D. Munblit. 2022. Risk factors for post-COVID-19 condition in previously hospitalised children using the ISARIC Global follow-up protocol: A prospective cohort study. *European Respiratory Journal* 59(2):2101341. https://doi.org/10.1183/13993003.01341-2021.

Parker, A. M., E. Brigham, B. Connolly, J. McPeake, A. V. Agranovich, M. T. Kenes, K. Casey, C. Reynolds, K. F. R. Schmidt, S. Y. Kim, A. Kaplin, C. M. Sevin, M. B. Brodsky, and A. E. Turnbull. 2021. Addressing the post-acute sequelae of SARS-CoV-2 infection: A multidisciplinary model of care. *Lancet Respiratory Medicine* 9(11):1328-1341. https://dx.doi.org/10.1016/s2213-2600(21)00385-4.

Petersen, M. S., M. F. Kristiansen, K. D. Hanusson, M. E. Danielsen, Á. S. B, S. Gaini, M. Strøm, and P. Weihe. 2021. Long COVID in the Faroe Islands: A longitudinal study among nonhospitalized patients. *Clinical Infectious Diseases* 73(11):e4058-e4063. https://doi.org/10.1093/cid/ciaa1792.

Philip, K. E. J., S. Buttery, P. Williams, B. Vijayakumar, J. Tonkin, A. Cumella, L. Renwick, L. Ogden, J. K. Quint, S. L. Johnston, M. I. Polkey, and N. S. Hopkinson. 2022. Impact of COVID-19 on people with asthma: A mixed methods analysis from a UK wide survey. *BMJ Open Respiratory Research* 9(1):e001056. https://dx.doi.org/10.1136/bmjresp-2021-001056.

Poyiadji, N., G. Shahin, D. Noujaim, M. Stone, S. Patel, and B. Griffith. 2020. COVID-19–associated acute hemorrhagic necrotizing encephalopathy: Imaging features. *Radiology* 296(2):E119-E120. https://dx.doi.org/10.1148/radiol.2020201187.

Puhan, M. A., J. Fehr, T. Ballouz, D. Menges, R. Kouyos, A. Trkola, and C. Münz. 2021. *Zurich Coronavirus Cohort: an observational study to determine long-term clinical outcomes and immune responses after coronavirus infection (COVID-19), assess the influence of virus genetics, and examine the spread of the coronavirus in the population of the Canton of Zurich, Switzerland.* https://www.isrctn.com/ISRCTN14990068 (accessed June 17, 2022).

Radtke, T., A. Ulyte, M. A. Puhan, and S. Kriemler. 2021. Long-term symptoms after SARS-CoV-2 infection in children and adolescents. *Journal of the American Medical Association* 326(9):869. https://dx.doi.org/10.1001/jama.2021.11880.

Rogers, J. P., E. Chesney, D. Oliver, T. A. Pollak, P. McGuire, P. Fusar-Poli, M. S. Zandi, G. Lewis, and A. S. David. 2020. Psychiatric and neuropsychiatric presentations associated with severe coronavirus infections: A systematic review and meta-analysis with comparison to the COVID-19 pandemic. *Lancet Psychiatry* 7(7):611-627. https://dx.doi.org/10.1016/s2215-0366(20)30203-0.

Royal Society. 2020. *Long Covid: What is it, and what is needed?* London, UK: The Royal Society. DES7217.

Say, D., N. Crawford, S. McNab, D. Wurzel, A. Steer, and S. Tosif. 2021. Post-acute COVID-19 outcomes in children with mild and asymptomatic disease. *Lancet Child and Adolescent Health* 5(6):e22-e23. https://dx.doi.org/10.1016/s2352-4642(21)00124-3.

Scheper-Hughes, N., and M. M. Lock. 1987. The mindful body: A prolegomenon to future work in medical anthropology. *Medical Anthropology Quarterly* 1(1):6-41. https://doi.org/10.1525/maq.1987.1.1.02a00020.

Selb, M., G. Stucki, J. Li, M. Mukaino, L. Li, F. Gimigliano, and ISPRM ClinFIT Task Force. 2021. Developing ClinFIT COVID-19: An initiative to scale up rehabilitation for COVID-19 patients and survivors across the care continuum. *Journal of the International Society of Physical and Rehabilitation Medicine* 4(4):174-183. https://doi.org/10.4103/JISPRM-000128.

Sheikh, J. I., and J. A. Yesavage. 1986. Geriatric Depression Scale (GDS): Recent evidence and development of a shorter version. *Clinical Gerontologist* 5(1-2):165-173. https://doi.org/10.1300/J018v05n01_09.

Singh, I., P. Joseph, P. M. Heerdt, M. Cullinan, D. D. Lutchmansingh, M. Gulati, J. D. Possick, D. M. Systrom, and A. B. Waxman. 2022. Persistent exertional intolerance after COVID-19: Insights from invasive cardiopulmonary exercise testing. *Chest* 161(1):54-63. https://pubmed.ncbi.nlm.nih.gov/34389297 (accessed June 15, 2022).

Spitzer, R. L., K. Kroenke, J. B. W. Williams, and B. Löwe. 2006. A brief measure for assessing generalized anxiety disorder. *Archives of Internal Medicine* 166(10):1092. https://dx.doi.org/10.1001/archinte.166.10.1092.

Stenton, C. 2008. The MRC breathlessness scale. *Occupational Medicine* 58(3):226-227. https://doi.org/10.1093/occmed/kqm162.

Stephenson, T., S. P. Pereira, R. Shafran, B. De Stavola, N. Rojas, K. McOwat, R. Simmons, M. Zavala, L. O'Mahoney, T. Chalder, E. Crawley, T. Ford, A. Harnden, I. Heyman, O. Swann, L. Whittaker, C. C. C. Consortium, and S. Ladhani. 2021 (unpublished). *Long COVID - the physical and mental health of children and non-hospitalised young people 3 months after SARS-CoV-2 infection; A national matched cohort study (the CLOCK) Study.* Research Square Platform LLC. https://doi.org/10.21203/rs.3.rs-798316/v1.

Sudre, C. H., B. Murray, T. Varsavsky, M. S. Graham, R. S. Penfold, R. C. Bowyer, J. C. Pujol, K. Klaser, M. Antonelli, L. S. Canas, E. Molteni, M. Modat, M. Jorge Cardoso, A. May, S. Ganesh, R. Davies, L. H. Nguyen, D. A. Drew, C. M. Astley, A. D. Joshi, J. Merino, N. Tsereteli, T. Fall, M. F. Gomez, E. L. Duncan, C. Menni, F. M. K. Williams, P. W. Franks, A. T. Chan, J. Wolf, S. Ourselin, T. Spector, and C. J. Steves. 2021. Attributes and predictors of long COVID. *Nature Medicine* 27(4):626-631. https://dx.doi.org/10.1038/s41591-021-01292-y.

Tabacof, L., J. Tosto-Mancuso, J. Wood, M. Cortes, A. Kontorovich, D. McCarthy, D. Rizk, G. Rozanski, E. Breyman, L. Nasr, C. Kellner, J. E. Herrera, and D. Putrino. 2022. Post-acute COVID-19 syndrome negatively impacts physical function, cognitive function, health-related quality of life, and participation. *American Journal of Physical Medicine & Rehabilitation* 101(1):48-52. https://doi.org/10.1097/PHM.0000000000001910.

Taquet, M., J. R. Geddes, M. Husain, S. Luciano, and P. J. Harrison. 2021. 6-month neurological and psychiatric outcomes in 236,379 survivors of COVID-19: A retrospective cohort study using electronic health records. *Lancet Psychiatry* 8(5):416-427. https://dx.doi.org/10.1016/s2215-0366(21)00084-5.

Townsend, L., A. H. Dyer, K. Jones, J. Dunne, A. Mooney, F. Gaffney, L. O'Connor, D. Leavy, K. O'Brien, J. Dowds, J. A. Sugrue, D. Hopkins, I. Martin-Loeches, C. Ni Cheallaigh, P. Nadarajan, A. M. McLaughlin, N. M. Bourke, C. Bergin, C. O'Farrelly, C. Bannan, and N. Conlon. 2020. Persistent fatigue following SARS-CoV-2 infection is common and independent of severity of initial infection. *PLOS ONE* 15(11):e0240784. https://dx.doi.org/10.1371/journal.pone.0240784.

UK CIS (United Kingdom Coronavirus Infection Survey). 2021. *Updated estimates of the prevalence of long COVID symptoms.* https://www.ons.gov.uk/peoplepopulationandcommunity/healthandsocialcare/healthandlifeexpectancies/adhocs/12788updatedestimatesoftheprevalenceoflongcovidsymptoms (accessed June 17, 2022).

Üstün, T. B., N. Kostanjesek, S. Chatterji, J. Rehm, and World Health Organization (Eds.). 2010. Measuring health and disability: Manual for WHO Disability Assessment Schedule (WHODAS 2.0). Geneva, Switzerland: World Health Organization. https://apps.who.int/iris/handle/10665/43974/ (accessed May 11, 2022).

Van Geelen, S. M., R. J. Bakker, W. Kuis, and E. M. Van De Putte. 2010. Adolescent chronic fatigue syndrome. *Archives of Pediatrics and Adolescent Medicine* 164(9). https://dx.doi.org/10.1001/archpediatrics.2010.145.

Viola, P., M. Ralli, D. Pisani, D. Malanga, D. Sculco, L. Messina, C. Laria, T. Aragona, G. Leopardi, F. Ursini, A. Scarpa, D. Topazio, A. Cama, V. Vespertini, F. Quintieri, L. Cosco, E. M. Cunsolo, and G. Chiarella. 2021. Tinnitus and equilibrium disorders in COVID-19 patients: Preliminary results. *European Archives of Oto-Rhino-Laryngology* 278(10):3725-3730. https://dx.doi.org/10.1007/s00405-020-06440-7.

Wasilewski, M. B., S. R. Cimino, K. M. Kokorelias, R. Simpson, S. L. Hitzig, and L. Robinson. 2022. Providing rehabilitation to patients recovering from COVID-19: A scoping review. *PM&R* 14(2):239-258. https://doi.org/10.1002/pmrj.12669.

Whitaker, M., J. Elliott, M. Chadeau-Hyam, S. Riley, A. Darzi, G. Cooke, H. Ward, and P. Elliott. 2021. *Persistent symptoms following SARS-CoV-2 infection in a random community sample of 508,707 people.* MedRxiv. https://doi.org/10.1101/2021.06.28.21259452.

WHO (World Health Organization). 2001. *ICF: International classification of functioning, disability and health.* Geneva, Switzerland: World Health Organization. https://apps.who.int/iris/bitstream/handle/10665/42407/9241545429.pdf;jsessionid=0E572EB55 5ED484EE7A789387FCF7DD8?sequence=1 (accessed June 15, 2022).

WHO. 2021. *A clinical case definition of post COVID-19 condition by a Delphi consensus.* Geneva, Switzerland: World Health Organization. https://www.who.int/publications/i/item/WHO-2019-nCoV-Post_COVID-19_condition-Clinical_case_definition-2021.1/ (accessed May 11, 2022).

Wiertz, C. M. H., W. A. J. Vints, G. J. C. M. Maas, S. M. C. Rasquin, Y. Y. van Horn, M. P. M. Dremmen, B. Hemmen, and J. A. Verbunt. 2021. COVID-19: Patient characteristics in the first phase of postintensive care rehabilitation. *Archives of Rehabilitation Research and Clinical Translation* 3(2):100108-100108. https://doi.org/10.1016/j.arrct.2021.100108.

Williams, N. 2017. The MRC breathlessness scale. *Occupational Medicine* 67(6):496-497. https://doi.org/10.1093/occmed/kqx086.

Wu, X., X. Liu, Y. Zhou, H. Yu, R. Li, Q. Zhan, F. Ni, S. Fang, Y. Lu, X. Ding, H. Liu, R. M. Ewing, M. G. Jones, Y. Hu, H. Nie, and Y. Wang. 2021. 3-month, 6-month, 9-month, and 12-month respiratory outcomes in patients following COVID-19-related hospitalisation: A prospective study. *Lancet Respiratory Medicine* 9(7):747-754. https://dx.doi.org/10.1016/s2213-2600(21)00174-0.

Zimmermann, P., L. F. Pittet, and N. Curtis. 2021. How common is long COVID in children and adolescents? *Pediatric Infectious Disease Journal* 40(12):e482-e487. https://doi.org/10.1097/INF.0000000000003328.

Appendix B

Workshop Agenda

Monday, March 21, 2022
Eastern Daylight Time

10:30 a.m. **Welcome and Workshop Overview**
WALTER R. FRONTERA, University of Puerto Rico School of Medicine
Workshop Planning Committee Chair

Sponsor Remarks from the Social Security Administration
STEVE ROLLINS, Acting Associate Commissioner, Office of Disability Policy, Social Security Administration
VINCENT NIBALI, Policy Analyst, Office of Medical Policy, Office of Disability Policy, Social Security Administration

10:50 a.m. **Session 1: Overview of Long COVID and Disability**

Moderator:
WALTER R. FRONTERA, University of Puerto Rico School of Medicine

What Is Long COVID?
STUART KATZ, NYU Langone Health

Long COVID and the Burden of Disease
THEO VOS, University of Washington, and SARAH WULF
    HANSON, University of Washington

**Pandemic-Related Effects on Work and the U.S.
Labor Force**
RAKESH KOCHHAR, Pew Research Center

Panel Discussion

12:15 p.m.   **Lunch Break**

1:00 p.m.   **Session 2: Postacute Sequelae of SARS-CoV-2 Infection
               and Implications for Recovery**

Moderator:
STEVEN DEEKS, University of California, San Francisco

Neurological and Neuromuscular Sequelae
AVINDRA NATH, National Institute of Neurological Disorders
    and Stroke, National Institutes of Health

Neuropsychiatric Sequelae
EMILY TROYER, University of California, San Diego

Cardiovascular Sequelae and Autonomic Syndrome
PETER NOVAK, Brigham and Women's Hospital

Pulmonary Sequelae
ANN MARIE PARKER, Johns Hopkins Medicine

Musculoskeletal, Fatigue, and Pain Sequelae
ANTHONY KOMAROFF, Brigham and Women's Hospital

Panel Discussion

2:30 p.m.   **Break**

2:45 p.m.	**Session 3: Patient and Caregiver Perspectives on Living with Long COVID** *Moderator:* MANSOOR MALIK, Johns Hopkins University School of Medicine Participants: - ANGELA MERIQUEZ VÁZQUEZ - JUAN LEWIS - LUCAS DENAULT AND KARIN DENAULT - TREVA TAYLOR **Panel Discussion**
3:50 p.m.	**Closing Remarks** WALTER R. FRONTERA, University of Puerto Rico School of Medicine Workshop Planning Committee Chair
4:00 p.m.	**Adjourn Day 1**

Tuesday, March 22, 2022
Eastern Daylight Time

10:30 a.m.	**Welcome and Day 2 Overview** WALTER R. FRONTERA, University of Puerto Rico School of Medicine Workshop Planning Committee Chair
10:35 a.m.	**Session 4: Long-Term Impairments and Functional Limitations Related to Long COVID** *Moderator:* LAURA MALONE, Kennedy Krieger Institute **ClinFIT COVID-19: A Functioning-Based Tool for Clinical Practice and Research** GEROLD STUCKI, University of Lucerne

Long-Term Functional Limitations Related to Long COVID in Adults
LAURA TABACOF, Mount Sinai

Functional Limitations and Impairments After COVID-19 ICU Stay
ALBA MIRANDA AZOLA, Johns Hopkins Medicine

Long-COVID and Mental Health Effects
MONICA KURYLO, University of Kansas Medical Center

Considerations in Child and Adolescent Functioning
ALICIA JOHNSTON, Boston Children's Hospital

Panel Discussion

12:00 p.m.   Lunch Break

12:45 p.m.   **Session 5: Clinical Practices and System Approaches for Improving Health and Recovery from Long COVID**

Moderator:
MONICA VERDUZCO-GUTIERREZ, UT Health San Antonio

Clinical Guidance Statements
STEVEN FLANAGAN, NYU-Langone Health

Integrated Care Models for Treating Adults and Children
BENJAMIN ABRAMOFF, University of Pennsylvania
AMANDA MORROW, Kennedy Krieger Institute

Overcoming Barriers to Health and Social Inequities in Long COVID Care
ZACKARY BERGER, Johns Hopkins Medicine

Panel Discussion

2:05 p.m.   Break

2:15 p.m.	**Session 6: Future Directions in the Treatment of Long COVID**
	Moderator: ANDREA LERNER, National Institute of Allergy and Infectious Diseases, National Institutes of Health
	Emerging Therapies STEVEN DEEKS, University of California, San Francisco
	Panel Discussion
	Panelists: • STEVEN DEEKS, University of California, San Francisco • WALTER R. FRONTERA, University of Puerto Rico School of Medicine • AVINDRA NATH, National Institute of Neurological Disorders and Stroke, National Institutes of Health
3:00 p.m.	**Closing Remarks** WALTER R. FRONTERA, University of Puerto Rico School of Medicine Workshop Planning Committee Chair
3:15 p.m.	**Adjourn Workshop**

Appendix C

Biographical Sketches of Workshop Planning Committee Members and Speakers

PLANNING COMMITTEE[1]

Walter R. Frontera, M.D., Ph.D., FRCP (*Chair*),* is professor of physical medicine and rehabilitation and physiology at the University of Puerto Rico School of Medicine. He formerly served as inaugural chair and professor of physical medicine and rehabilitation at Harvard Medical School and Vanderbilt University School of Medicine. Dr. Frontera's main research interest is the mechanisms underlying muscle atrophy and weakness in the elderly, and the development of rehabilitative interventions for sarcopenia. He is editor in chief of the *American Journal of Physical Medicine and Rehabilitation* and the immediate past president of the International Society of Physical and Rehabilitation Medicine. Dr. Frontera received his medical degree from the University of Puerto Rico School of Medicine and a Ph.D. in applied anatomy and physiology from Boston University. He is a member of the National Academy of Medicine and has served on numerous National Academies' committees, including the Standing Committee of Medical and Vocational Experts for the Social Security Administration's Disability Programs, the Committee on the Use of Selected Assistive Products and Technologies in Eliminating or Reducing the Effects of Impairments, and the Planning Committee on Long-Term Health Effects Stemming from COVID-19 and Implications for the Social

---

[1] Planning committee members marked with an asterisk also served as speakers or moderators at the workshop.

Security Administration. Dr. Frontera is also a fellow of the Royal College of Physicians in London.

Adaora A. Adimora, M.D., M.P.H., is Sarah Graham Kenan Distinguished Professor of Medicine and professor of epidemiology at the University of North Carolina at Chapel Hill. She is an internist who subspecializes in infectious diseases. Her research interest is the clinical and social epidemiology of HIV and other sexually transmitted infections with a focus on minority populations. She is a member of the National Institutes of Health COVID Treatment Guidelines Panel. Dr. Adimora is a fellow of the American College of Physicians and the Infectious Diseases Society of America (IDSA). She was recently elected to the IDSA Board of Directors and is a member of the National Academy of Medicine. She earned her M.D. from the Yale School of Medicine and an M.P.H. in Epidemiology from the UNC Gillings School of Global Public Health. She did her residency in Internal Medicine at Boston City Hospital and Infectious Diseases fellowship at Montefiore/Albert Einstein.

Rany Condos, M.D., is professor of clinical medicine in the Division of Pulmonary and Critical Care Medicine at NYU Langone Health. She is director of the Adult Cystic Fibrosis program and heads the Advanced Lung Diseases program at NYU. She serves on the Data Safety Monitoring Board for the Cystic Fibrosis Foundation. Her recent charge has been as program director of the post-COVID clinical program at NYU. Dr. Condos is currently the principal investigator of a multicenter NIAID-funded study of a treatment to mitigate post-COVID fibrosis. Her research interests include targeted immunomodulation in lung disease, and she holds a patent for the use of inhaled interferon gamma in the treatment of lung disease including idiopathic pulmonary fibrosis and tuberculosis.

Steven G. Deeks, M.D.,* is professor of medicine in residence at the University of California, San Francisco. He is a recognized expert on the effect of HIV and other viral infections on inflammation, immune function, and health. Dr. Deeks has published over 600 peer-reviewed articles, editorials, and invited reviews on these and related topics. He has been the recipient of several National Institutes of Health (NIH) grants, and is one of the principal investigators of the Delaney AIDS Research Enterprise, which is an NIH-funded international collaboratory aimed at developing therapeutic interventions to cure HIV infection. He is also the principal investigator of amfAR Institute for HIV Cure Research. In March, 2020, he used his HIV research program to construct the "Long-term Impact of Infection with Novel Coronavirus" cohort, which is now supporting dozens of studies addressing the effects of

SARS-CoV-2 on health. He was elected to the American Society for Clinical Investigation and the Association of America Physicians. He is editor-in-chief for *Current Opinion in HIV and AIDS* and serves on the scientific advisory board for *Science Translational Medicine*. In addition to his clinical and translational investigation, Dr. Deeks maintains a primary care clinic for people living with HIV.

Andrea M. Lerner, M.D., M.S.,* is an infectious diseases physician and medical officer in the Office of the Director of the National Institute of Allergy and Infectious Diseases (NIAID), of the National Institutes of Health. In her current role, Dr. Lerner supports the NIAID Director and NIAID mission on a broad range of issues related to infectious diseases and public health, including leading the organization of the virtual Workshop on Post-Acute Sequelae of COVID-19 in December, 2020. Lerner also serves as an attending physician in the NIH Clinical Center on the NIH Clinical Infectious Diseases Consult Service. She is board certified in Internal Medicine and Infectious Diseases by the American Board of Internal Medicine and is a member of the Infectious Diseases Society of America. She earned her medical degree from George Washington University in Washington, D.C., and completed internal medicine internship and residency training at Thomas Jefferson University in Philadelphia, Pennsylvania. Following residency training, Dr. Lerner practiced as a hospitalist physician in San Diego and Baltimore before completing her fellowship in infectious diseases at NIAID.

Mansoor A. Malik, M.D., M.B.A., M.B.B.S.,* is clinical professor of psychiatry at Johns Hopkins University School of Medicine. He has previously served as professor and residency program director at Howard University Hospital for over 10 years, where he trained and mentored over 100 minority residents and medical students. He has received multiple teaching and professional awards for his services. He previously served as president of Washington Psychiatry Society, one of the oldest and most prestigious mental health organizations in the country. He has also been elected to the American College of Psychiatrists, one of the highest honors for a psychiatrist in the United States. He completed his medical training at Rawalpindi Medical College in 1995 and completed Membership of Royal College of Psychiatrists before moving to the United States.

Laura A. Malone, M.D., Ph.D.,* is a pediatric neurologist and codirector of the Pediatric Post-COVID-19 Rehabilitation Clinic at the Kennedy Krieger Institute in Baltimore, Maryland. She is also a physician scientist in the Center for Movement Studies and assistant professor of neurology and physical medicine and rehabilitation at the Johns Hopkins University School of Medicine.

Dr. Malone addresses the pediatric neurology needs of children with postacute or Long COVID syndromes and is actively engaged in research to improve outcomes for children after COVID-19. Her research interests also include neurorehabilitation and improving outcomes after neurological injury. She coleads the Pediatric Working Group on the American Academy of Physical Medicine and Rehabilitation's Long COVID/PASC Quality Improvement Collaborative, which is an interdisciplinary group of experts working on developing guidance statements for the treatment of Long COVID. In 2020, Dr. Malone was awarded the Frank L. Coulson, Jr., Award for Clinical Excellence and in 2018 was inducted into the Distinguished Teaching Society at the Johns Hopkins School of Medicine. She is a member of the International Pediatric Rehabilitation Collaborative, the Child Neurology Society, as well as numerous other professional societies related to neurological rehabilitation. Dr. Malone has a Ph.D. in biomedical engineering from the Johns Hopkins School of Medicine where she studied gait rehabilitation and motor control after brain injury. She earned her M.D. from the University of North Carolina at Chapel Hill and completed her residency in pediatrics and pediatric neurology at Johns Hopkins Hospital.

Avindra Nath, M.D.,* is clinical director of the National Institute of Neurological Disorders and Stroke (NINDS) at the National Institutes of Health, where he is also chief of the Section of Infections of the Nervous System and director of the Translational Center for Neurological Sciences. Dr. Avindra Nath is a physician–scientist who specializes in neuroimmunology and neurovirology. His research is focused on the clinical manifestations, pathophysiology, and treatment of emerging neurological infections with a focus on HIV infection. In recent years, he has studied the neurological complications of endogenous retroviruses, Ebola, Zika virus, and SARS-CoV-2 and conducts research on patients with undiagnosed neuroinflammatory disorders. He has served on advisory committees to NIH, the Centers for Disease Control and Prevention, the U.S. Food and Drug Administration, and the World Health Organization. The International Society of NeuroVirology gave him the Pioneer in NeuroVirology Award for his contributions to HIV neuropathogenesis and elected him as the president of the society. He received the Wybran award from the Society of Neuroimmune Pharmacology for contributions to neurovirology. He also received the NIH Director's award for his work on SARS-CoV-2 and the Health and Human Services Secretary's award for his work on Ebola infection.

Monica Verduzco-Gutierrez, M.D.,* is an accomplished academic physiatrist, and professor and chair of the Department of Rehabilitation Medicine at the Joe R. and Teresa Lozano Long School of Medicine at UT Health in San

Antonio, Texas. She previously was medical director of the Brain Injury and Stroke Program at TIRR Memorial Hermann Hospital, a top two *U.S. News and World Report* Best Hospital for Rehabilitation. She is currently clinical chief of physical medicine and rehabilitation at the University Hospital System, and medical director of Critical Illness Recovery and Neurorehabilitation at Warm Springs Rehabilitation Hospitals in San Antonio, Texas. Her area of clinical expertise is the care of patients with traumatic brain injury, stroke rehabilitation, and interventional spasticity management. She is currently directing COVID-19 Recovery Clinics, the first in south Texas, which aligns with her mission to increase access to interdisciplinary care, optimize function, and improve quality of life for survivors with Long COVID. Dr. Gutierrez is a passionate advocate for physiatry and for underrepresented groups in medicine via social media channels. She is the social media editor of the *American Journal of Physical Medicine and Rehabilitation*. She is on the board of trustees of the Association of Academic Physiatrists. In 2019, she received the Top 25 Women in Healthcare Award from the National Diversity Council and Healthcare Diversity Council, which recognizes the top women leaders in the city of Houston.

WORKSHOP SPEAKERS

Benjamin Abramoff, M.D., M.S., is assistant professor of physical medicine and rehabilitation medicine at the University of Pennsylvania. He founded and directs the Penn Medicine COVID assessment and Recovery Clinic, one of the first comprehensive clinics for post-COVID care in the country. To date, the clinic has treated over 1,200 patients with persistent symptoms following acute COVID infections. Considered a national expert, he wrote the widely referred to *UpToDate Post-COVID Guidelines*. He also serves as cochair of the American Academy of Physical Medicine and Rehabilitation (AAPM&R) Post-COVID Clinic Collaborative, which has developed clinical consensus guidelines on post-COVID syndrome care. He has advised the Centers for Disease Control and Prevention, the National Institutes of Health, and the National Council on Disability on post-COVID issues.

Alba Azola, M.D., is a rehabilitation physician helping patients restore function and movement after an injury or illness. She is codirector of the Post-Acute COVID Team at Johns Hopkins Hospital, a multidisciplinary clinic for patients with lingering symptoms after SARS-CoV-2 infection. Dr. Azola completed her residency in physical medicine and rehabilitation at the Johns Hopkins Department of Physical Medicine and Rehabilitation, where in her final year she was awarded the Frank L. Coulson, Jr., Award for Clinical Excellence.

Zackary Berger, M.D., Ph.D., FACP, is associate professor in the Division of General Internal Medicine at the Johns Hopkins School of Medicine, as well as in the Johns Hopkins School of Public Health, and core faculty at the Johns Hopkins Berman Institute of Bioethics. He maintains an active internal medicine practice in Baltimore both at Johns Hopkins and at the Esperanza Center Health Clinic, where, as staff physician, he cares for undocumented immigrants. He has published widely on shared decision making, bioethics, and health justice. He is currently involved in two ethnographic projects regarding the experience of the COVID pandemic on the part of two groups: Latinx in Baltimore and Charedim in New York. His latest work, an edited volume of essays on progressive health care entitled *Health for Everyone*, is in press, and he is currently thinking and reading about solidarity-based health care outside of government control.

Lucas Denault, joined by his mother, **Karin Denault,** a working mother of four, is a 16-year-old high school junior from South Central Pennsylvania. Prior to becoming positive for COVID-19 in January of 2021, Lucas was a highly functioning student and varsity athlete. Since the onset of Long COVID, Lucas has been a patient of the Kennedy Krieger Institute Post-COVID-19 Rehabilitation Clinic.

Steven R. Flanagan, M.D., is highly recognized, nationally and internationally, as one of the leading experts in the area of brain injury rehabilitation. Dr. Steven Flanagan joined NYU Langone Health and the NYU Grossman School of Medicine in 2008 as professor and chair of rehabilitation medicine and medical director of Rusk Rehabilitation. He previously served as vice chairman of rehabilitation medicine at Mount Sinai School of Medicine. He serves on several national and international medical advisory boards as well as the editorial board for the *Journal of Head Trauma Rehabilitation*. He served in multiple leadership roles for the American Academy of Physical Medicine and Rehabilitation where he is currently vice president. He authored numerous chapters and peer-reviewed publications, and participated in both federally and industry-sponsored research. He served as panel chair for several national review panels including the Veterans Administration and the Congressionally Directed Medical Research Program—Department of Defense program for traumatic brain injury. Dr. Flanagan has received awards for his work as an educator, clinician, and advocate for people with brain injury from several organizations, including the Brain Injury Association of New York State, Mount Sinai Medical Center, Brain Injury Assistance, North American Brain Injury Association, and Rutgers—New Jersey Medical School. Castle Connolly has continually listed him as one of America's Top Doctors since 2010.

Sarah Wulf Hanson, M.P.H., Ph.D., is a research scientist at the Institute for Health Metrics and Evaluation (IHME) at the University of Washington. She has more than a decade of experience estimating the burden of disease of several diseases, conditions, and risk factors in the Global Burden of Disease (GBD) study. In her current role, she is working to improve the GBD methods and the stability of estimates over time, as well as estimating the health burden of acute and Long COVID disability. Dr. Hanson received both her M.P.H. and Ph.D. in global health metrics from the University of Washington, after receiving a B.S. in bioengineering from Rice University.

Alicia Johnston, M.D., received her M.D. from SUNY Upstate Medical University and completed her pediatric residency and fellowship in infectious diseases at Duke University Medical Center. She is currently an instructor at Harvard Medical School and an attending physician in the Division of Infectious Diseases at Boston Children's Hospital where she codirects the Multidisciplinary Post-COVID-19 Program.

Stuart D. Katz, M.D., M.S., is Helen L. and Martin S. Kimmel Professor of Advanced Cardiac Therapeutics and contact principal investigator for the RECOVER Clinical Science Core at New York University Langone Health. He is also chair of the NYU Grossman School of Medicine IRB Board B and chair of the NYU CTSI expanded Scientific Review Committee. Dr. Katz's academic pursuits have been devoted to clinical care and research in cardiovascular diseases for more than 30 years. Dr. Katz has received continuous research funding from the NIH for the last 30 years, has authored more than 200 original research contributions, review articles, books, and book chapters on heart failure, vascular physiology, exercise physiology, and clinical pharmacology.

Rakesh Kochhar, Ph.D., is senior researcher at Pew Research Center. He is an expert on trends in employment, income, and wealth. His research has focused on the American and global middle classes and the economic well-being of White, Black, Hispanic, Asian, and immigrant workers. Prior to joining Pew Research Center, he was senior economist at Joel Popkin and Company, where he served as a consultant to government agencies, private firms, international agencies, and labor unions. Kochhar received his doctorate in economics from Brown University. He has appeared on numerous media outlets, including NPR, CNN, MSNBC, and Fox News. He has testified before Congress and regularly speaks at professional, academic, and business conferences.

Anthony L. Komaroff, M.D., is Steven P. Simcox/Patrick A. Clifford/James H. Higby Professor of Medicine at Harvard Medical School, senior physician at Brigham and Women's Hospital in Boston, and editor in chief of the *Harvard Health Letter*. He was director of the division of general medicine and primary care at Brigham and Women's Hospital for 15 years, and is the founding editor of *Journal Watch*, a summary medical information newsletter for physicians published by the Massachusetts Medical Society/New England Journal of Medicine.

Monica Kurylo, Ph.D., ABPP, is professor and director of the Division of Psychology in the Department of Psychiatry and Behavioral Sciences at the University of Kansas Medical Center (KUMC). Dr. Kurylo, who joined the faculty in 2005, has appointments in both the Department of Psychiatry and Behavioral Sciences and the Department of Rehabilitation Medicine. She also is director of neurorehabilitation psychology at the University of Kansas Health System. In addition to receiving her doctorate degree in clinical psychology (health/rehabilitation emphases) at the University of Kansas, Dr. Kurylo has internship and postdoctoral experience in rehabilitation psychology and neuropsychology. She is board certified in rehabilitation psychology through the American Board of Professional Psychology (ABPP). Dr. Kurylo leads the psychology division in the Department of Psychiatry, which includes a team of 19 psychologists in both inpatient and outpatient settings throughout the medical center and KU Hospital. As director of neurorehabilitation psychology services and program director for the neurorehabilitation psychology fellowship at KU Medical Center, Dr. Kurylo provides inpatient and outpatient evaluation and treatment services as well as consults as a member of the interdisciplinary treatment teams in rehabilitation, burn, and trauma. Dr. Kurylo is codirector for the KU-Lawrence health psychology major and leadership team coordinator/primary supervisor for the health psychology practicum at KU Medical Center for the KU-Lawrence clinical psychology graduate students. She is vice chair of the Appointments, Promotions, and Tenure Committee in the KU School of Medicine, and a member of the Promotions and Tenure Committees for both psychiatry and rehabilitation medicine departments in Kansas City. She is a representative from Division 22 (Rehabilitation Psychology) to the American Psychological Association (APA) Council of Representatives, a member of the APA Health Care Financing Advisory group, and a representative to the Interdivisional Healthcare Council for Division 31 (State, Provincial and Territorial Psychology Affairs). She is a neuropsychologist consultant for concussion/traumatic brain injury and cancer research at KUMC. Dr. Kurylo is a member of the KU Health System Long-COVID clinic and the AAPM&R PASC Multidisciplinary Quality Improvement Initiative Collaborative (KU Health System) in which she serves as clinical lead for the Mental Health and Neuropsychiatric Symptoms in Patients with PASC Consensus Guidance.

Juan "Lou" Lewis lives in San Antonio, Texas, and is a veteran of the U.S armed forces. Lewis became ill with COVID-19 in April 2020 while working abroad.

Amanda Morrow, M.D., is assistant professor in the Johns Hopkins Department of Physical Medicine and Rehabilitation specializing in pediatric rehabilitation medicine. She sees patients at Mt. Washington Pediatric Hospital, Kennedy Krieger Institute, and the Johns Hopkins Children's Center. Her clinical practice focuses on maximizing the functional potential of children with congenital and acquired disabilities. Dr. Morrow is codirector of the Pediatric Post COVID-19 Rehabilitation Clinic at Kennedy Krieger Institute. Dr. Morrow received her medical degree at the University of Pittsburgh School of Medicine and went on to complete her residency in physical medicine and rehabilitation at Sinai Hospital in Baltimore, where she served as chief resident. She then completed her fellowship in pediatric rehabilitation medicine at the Johns Hopkins Hospital/Kennedy Krieger Institute. Her research has focused on the use of diagnostic tests to aid in rehabilitation management for children with complex medical needs and examining the effects of caregiver concerns on medication adherence in complex patient populations. She is involved in the national quality improvement collaborative for Long COVID/Post-Acute Sequelae of SARS-CoV-2 infection (PASC) through the American Academy of Physical Medicine and Rehabilitation and is currently focusing her research efforts on Long COVID in children.

Peter Novak, M.D., Ph.D., is director of the Autonomic Laboratory at Brigham and Women's Hospital. He is a board-certified neurologist and a board-certified autonomic specialist. He is a member of American Academy of Neurology, American Autonomic Society, and a member of Autonomic Board of the United Council for Neurologic Subspecialties (UCNS). He graduated from medical school in Bratislava, Slovakia, and completed his neurology residency at the Ohio State University. He also completed postdoctoral studies focusing on cardiovascular and autonomic research at Charles University (Prague), University of Montreal, McGill University (Montreal), and Mayo Clinic. He has special interests in autoimmune, small fiber, and autonomic neuropathies associated with COVID-19 and Lyme disease, postural tachycardia syndrome (POTS), and multiple system atrophy. He has written more than 80 papers and presented at numerous conferences.

Ann M. Parker, M.D., Ph.D., is an intensivist and assistant professor in the Division of Pulmonary and Critical Care Medicine at Johns Hopkins. Dr. Parker completed a residency in internal medicine at the University of Maryland Medical Center and a fellowship in pulmonary and critical care medicine at the Johns Hopkins Hospital. She obtained her Ph.D. in clinical investigation at the Johns Hopkins University Bloomberg School of Public Health. Her research over the last decade has focused on understanding and improving outcomes for survivors of critical illness. Dr. Parker is principal investigator on an NIH-funded randomized controlled trial evaluating an intervention to improve depression symptoms and physical function among survivors of acute respiratory failure. Over the last 2 years, she has applied her expertise in critical illness outcomes to address the needs of COVID-19 survivors as cofounder and codirector of the Johns Hopkins Post-Acute COVID-19 Team (PACT) Program. She has also served as a member of working groups with the NIH and World Health Organization (WHO) to identify key research priorities for postacute sequelae of SARS-CoV-2.

Gerold Stucki, M.D., M.S., is professor and chair of the Department of Health Sciences and Medicine at the University of Lucerne, founder and director of the Center for Rehabilitation in Global Health Systems—a WHO Collaborating Center at the same university, and director of Swiss Paraplegic Research in Nottwil, Switzerland. After his medical studies and his clinical training in physical and rehabilitation medicine and rheumatology, he obtained a master of science in health policy and management from the Harvard School of Public Health and a diploma in biostatistics and epidemiology from the University of McGill. In 2013, he was appointed foreign associate of the U.S. National Academy of Medicine, and since 2018 he has been acting as vice president of the European Academy of Rehabilitation Medicine. Dr. Stucki has authored more than 600 publications.

Laura Tabacof, M.D., is a specialist in physical medicine and rehabilitation. As research instructor at the Department of Rehabilitation and Human Performance at Icahn School of Medicine at Mount Sinai, Dr. Tabacof has been developing novel rehabilitation approaches and spearheading research of Long COVID-19 biomarkers and quantifying impairment. Dr. Tabacof also serves as an active member of the WHO and AAPMR guidance development groups for Long COVID rehabilitation.

Treva M. Taylor previously served as assistant director of hospital risk management for Jacobi Medical Center, New York City Health and Hospitals Corporation. Taylor tested positive for COVID-19 in January 2021 and was hospitalized in the ICU at NYU Langone Health for 6 weeks.

Emily A. Troyer, M.D., is the child and adolescent psychiatry track director for the Community Psychiatry Program and NIMH T32 postdoctoral fellow in biological psychiatry and neuroscience in the Department of Psychiatry at the University of California, San Diego (UCSD). She completed residency training in general psychiatry at the University of Illinois at Chicago and child and adolescent psychiatry fellowship training at UCSD. In her current position as postdoctoral fellow, Dr. Troyer's primary research focuses on examining immunologic mechanisms in pediatric obsessive-compulsive disorder, under the mentorship of Dr. Suzi Hong and Dr. David Rosenberg. As a member of the Hong Laboratory, Dr. Troyer is also involved in broader projects related to immune and endocrine mechanisms underlying neuropsychiatric symptoms in the context of medical comorbidities such as obesity and hypertension in adults. Since the beginning of the COVID-19 pandemic, Dr. Troyer and colleagues have also investigated potential immunologic mechanisms in post-COVID neuropsychiatric symptoms.

Angela M. Vázquez, M.S.W., has spent nearly a decade in public policy, coalition building, and activism on behalf of children and families. Her work has been centered on ensuring the well-being of marginalized youth from birth through young adulthood, especially as their life opportunities are affected by their race, ethnicity, trauma, and poverty. Vázquez has spent the last decade in education and child welfare public policy, convening local and statewide education and child welfare stakeholders, and facilitating policy development and implementation discussions for children in foster care as policy analyst at Advancement Project and as associate director for FosterEd California. Currently, Vázquez is policy director at the Children's Partnership, covering a portfolio that includes mental health and child welfare, and she recently was appointed to California's Citizens Redistricting Commission, an independent body tasked with redrawing California's elections boundaries. In March 2020, Vázquez became ill with COVID-19 and has since developed Long COVID—a condition marked by prolonged, debilitating, relapsing-remitting symptoms experienced by up to one third of COVID-19 patients. As the president of Body Politic, an all-volunteer grassroots organization at the forefront of Long COVID patient advocacy, Vázquez is using her skills in leading intersectional health and well-being advocacy to advocate with and on behalf of other patients of color with postinfection chronic illness and disabilities. She received her masters degree in social work with honors in community organizing, planning, and administration from the University of Southern California after graduating cum laude from Claremont McKenna College with a B.A. in psychology. She also serves on the Board of Trustees at Pacific Oaks College in Pasadena.

Theo Vos, M.D., M.Sc., Ph.D., is professor of health metrics sciences at the Institute for Health Metrics and Evaluation (IHME) at the University of Washington. He is a key member of the research team for the landmark Global Burden of Disease (GBD) study, which is coordinated by IHME. In this role, he is working to improve the GBD methods, update sources of data, and develop partnerships with countries and disease experts to produce GBD estimates that are most relevant to policy decision making. He is also focused on linking the epidemiological estimates from GBD to information on health expenditure and cost-effectiveness. Dr. Vos received his Ph.D. in epidemiology and health economics from Erasmus University and his medical degree from State University Groningen, both in the Netherlands. He also studied at the London School of Hygiene and Tropical Medicine, where he obtained an M.Sc. in public health in developing countries.